small changes
big results

small changes
big results

A 12-Week Action Plan
to a Better Life

Ellie Krieger, MS, RD

WITH KELLY JAMES-ENGER

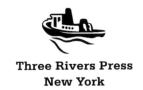

Three Rivers Press
New York

Grateful acknowledgment is made to Center for Science in the Public Interest for permission to reprint an excerpt from *Nutrition Action Healthletter.* Copyright © 2004 by CSPI. Reprinted by permission of Center for Science in the Public Interest, 1875 Connecticut Ave., NW., Suite 300, Washington, DC 20009-5728.

Published by Three Rivers Press, an imprint of the Crown Publishing Group, a division of Random House, Inc., New York.
www.crownpublishing.com

Three Rivers Press and the Tugboat design are registered trademarks of Random House, Inc.

Originally published in hardcover in the United States by Clarkson Potter/Publishers, an imprint of the Crown Publishing Group, a division of Random House, Inc., New York, in 2005.

Library of Congress Cataloging-in-Publication Data
Krieger, Ellie
    Small Changes, big results : a 12-week action plan to a better life / by Ellie Krieger, with Kelly James-Enger.
1. Health. 2. Physical fitness. 3. Nutrition. I. James-Enger, Kelly. II. Title.
    RA776.K6986 2005
    613.7-dc22   2004020126

ISBN-13: 9870-307-33587-6
ISBN-10: 0-307-33587-9

Printed in the United States of America

Design by Jane Treuhaft

10   9   8   7   6   5   4   3

for

thom

and

isabella

contents

introduction

Imagine yourself the best person you can be. You wake up each morning energized, feeling comfortable and confident in your body, moving with ease, and standing tall. Your life is full and exciting, yet you are grounded with a sense of balance. You are able to think fast and flow with life's challenges. You are surrounded by people you love, supported by them and supporting them in turn. And you know you are doing what you can to live a longer, healthier life.

You may feel this ideal is unattainable at times. But let me tell you something: you can be that person (or at least come close— you are human, after all!). All you have to do is make some small changes.

Most people I talk to *want* to look better, feel better, and live happier, more fulfilling lives. They may be motivated to make a change, but they're not sure what to do first—or they're overwhelmed by the idea of overhauling their entire lives. They get stuck before they even begin.

I know from working with hundreds of clients that the problem isn't lack of information—there's more data about nutrition, fitness, and wellness available than ever before. In fact, the opposite is true: we've become victims of information overload. Should you cut out red meat from your diet or keep it in? Increase your protein intake or slash your fat grams? Exercise seven days a week or only three? Lift weights or do yoga? We are bombarded by information every day, and it's nearly impossible to sort out what's helpful and valuable from some of the get-thin-quick schemes that almost never work.

I also see many people who want to change the way they eat and the way they treat their bodies, but they underestimate how difficult this kind of transformation can be. Or they bite off more than they can chew and try to change *everything* all at once. The problem is that they may not have the tools they need to change their lifestyle, or they become overwhelmed by trying to do too much, too soon.

Does this sound familiar? Well, I'm here to help you, and I've got good news: you *don't* have to overhaul your entire lifestyle or subject yourself to the latest fad diet. Making *small* changes is the key to transforming your life. By making small changes in your diet, activity level, and lifestyle, you can change the way you eat, move, and feel—without having to suffer, without needing expensive equipment or special foods, and without feeling overwhelmed.

When I work with clients, I take a three-pronged approach. I'm a dietitian, but I don't just focus on nutrition. This surprises many people, but I look at nutrition, fitness, and wellness as a three-legged stool. Each leg supports the others, and all are necessary for a balanced life.

In the chapters that follow, you'll learn how to make small changes in these three areas of your life. You'll be introduced to my 12-Week Action Plan that gives you all the tools you need to change your life. Each week sets out a specific change in the way you eat, the way you move, and the way you live and explains how to make the change as well as explaining why it will benefit you. By progressing in bite-sized chunks and building on what you did before, you'll find that eating, exercising, and living more healthfully is easier than you thought.

eating well

A lot of people want to lose weight, and my clients are always surprised that I don't put them on highly restrictive diets. When most people think about eating better or losing weight, they think about what to say "no" to. When you focus on what you *can't* have, it's no wonder you feel deprived and irritable! I take the opposite approach and concentrate instead on what you can say "yes" to.

Sure, there are foods you have to cut back on if you want to lose weight. Most of us can't down pizza and milkshakes all day without the extra calories showing up on our tummies or thighs. But food is not the enemy. Food is a wonderful, delicious, sensuous part of life, and it doesn't have to stop being so just because you're eating healthfully.

I help people discover all the great foods they can say "yes" to. When I talk about the "ideal" diet, I frame it in terms of what types of foods to eat rather than what foods to avoid. An ideal diet provides you with a wide variety of nutritious, delicious foods that you enjoy. It's a diet you can maintain because you like what you're eating, not a diet you have to force yourself to stick to. (See the Appendix for a sample week plan for a basic ideal diet.)

Don't confuse an "ideal" diet with a "perfect" diet. I tell clients frequently that there's no such thing as a perfect diet! In fact, people who constantly strive for the "perfect" diet usually obsess over food, which can be just as unhealthy and destructive as ignoring the way you eat.

There are no "bad" foods. But there *are* foods that you should eat rarely rather than all the time. You don't have to vow that you'll never eat chocolate cake again in order to revamp your eating. Instead of classifying foods as good or bad, I find it helps to categorize foods into three groups:

- **Usually:** these are foods you should base your diet on, and the foods you can always say "yes" to. Fruits, vegetables, whole grains, legumes, lean proteins, and low-fat and no-fat dairy products are all "Usually" foods.
- **Sometimes:** these are foods you can sometimes say "yes" to, like refined grains, higher-fat meats, and sugary foods.
- **Rarely:** these are foods that you should only rarely say "yes" to, like junk food, candy, fatty meats, and high-fat desserts. Yes, they can still be a part of your healthy diet. But they should be indulgences, not a daily thing. (For a full list of Usually/Sometimes/Rarely foods, see page 233.)

The nutritional component of my 12-Week Action Plan doesn't force you to suddenly change the way you're currently eating. Instead, you'll focus on one skill at a time, from learning the optimal timing for your meals to gradually incorporating the best foods into your life—the foods that will help keep you slim, healthy, and energized. There are also lots of recipes and tips along the way to give you all the tools you need to make the change successfully.

Finally, this is a way of eating, *not* a diet. As I see it, a diet is something you go on until you lose weight and then go off. It is a losing (or should I say regaining) mentality. To lose weight for good and to be optimally healthy, you need to make changes you can live with. My plan allows you to make small changes in the way you're eating now that will add up to better nutrition, more energy, and weight loss over the long haul.

moving your body

Eating well is only one part of the picture. You also have to be physically active to stay slim, feel your best, and live healthier. Many people moan and groan when I say this because they have been stuck on the sofa so long they have forgotten how good it actually feels to move.

Ask any dedicated exerciser why he or she does it, and answers will vary. "It helps me maintain my weight." "I can leave the stressors of the day behind at the gym." "Exercise gives me more energy." "It helps keep me healthy." But one of the most common reasons is a simple one—"It makes me feel good."

When you're in good physical shape, activity *does* feel good. Dancers, runners, yoga devotees, weight lifters, and even dedicated walkers all experience a mental and physical lift from exercise. This feeling, sometimes called a runner's high, creates an emotional boost and a positive sense of well-being.

Yet you needn't be a dedicated athlete to experience this joy of movement. Watch children playing: they run for the fun of it, jump in the air because it feels good. Somewhere between early childhood and teenage years, though, most of us begin to lose this experience, and settle down to a lifetime where we use our bodies only when we need them, which in our push-button world isn't very often.

But our bodies are meant to move! Just because modern life has become more sedentary doesn't mean we have to be. When exercise is a healthy habit, you'll notice a difference. You'll feel more energetic, more alert, and more alive. Regular exercise strengthens your immune system, builds stronger muscles and bones, and improves your cardiovascular health, reducing your risk of heart attacks and a slew of other conditions. It changes the way your body looks and the way you feel about your body—not just your physical appearance but your capabilities as well. It reduces anxiety, eases depression, and elevates mood.

If you haven't been in good physical shape since grade school, it can be tough getting started. I've found that most people have similar excuses (oops, I mean "reasons") when it comes to not exercising. "I don't have time!" is the number one reason; "I'm too tired" follows close on its heels. I think, though, that a major obstacle is people starting out usually don't exercise regularly enough for long enough so that it begins to feel good to them. They never get over the initial hump to make exercise a part of their life.

Many people start off aggressively and then find that the inevitable soreness and fatigue they experience provides them with the perfect excuse they need to give up exercise . . . until next year's New Year's resolutions roll around. But if you start off slowly and proceed gradually, you begin to see and feel the results, and those results become your incentive to make activity a priority. Let me tell you, I am not always gung-ho to work out. I sometimes drag myself to the gym or for a walk. But no matter how much I'd rather stay in bed, knowing from experience how a little exercise brings me to life and how it keeps me feeling good in my jeans somehow gets me going.

Even if you've been a dedicated couch potato for as long as you can remember, I'll help you make exercise happen in your own life. The fitness component of the

12-Week Action Plan is easy, doable, accessible, and well rounded. It includes all of the three elements of a comprehensive fitness program—strength, flexibility, and cardiovascular exercise.

I've made things easy by providing a program designed for anyone who hasn't exercised before or is coming back to working out after a long period of inactivity. (But as with any exercise program, please get your doctor's okay before you start.) If you're a regular exerciser, though, you can use this framework and then tweak it to make it challenging enough for you as well.

Best of all, you start at a level that's doable and build on what you've done before so that as your body becomes fitter, you're ready for each new step as the weeks go by. But moving more isn't only about exercising—it's about beginning to make movement a part of your life. I'll help you change your mindset and your approach so that you're leading an active life.

living well

The third component of the program is often overlooked by fitness-minded people. They realize it is important to eat better and move their bodies more, but they're surprised when I tell them there is one more key factor—to examine their lives to determine the biggest stressors, and figure out ways to reduce or eliminate them.

You can eat a nutritious diet and exercise regularly, but if you ignore your mental health and emotional well-being, you won't feel good. Learning how to reduce stress is an integral part of this program, as is mindfulness, which I'll discuss in a moment.

While stress has as many definitions as there are individuals, in medical terms it describes your body's response to events or actions that it perceives as threatening. You've probably heard of the "fight or flight" response: our ancestors had to be physiologically equipped to deal with stressors such as encountering a predator. When they sensed fear, their breathing and heart rate increased, and their heart pumped more blood to their muscles to prepare the body to respond. Hormones like adrenaline were produced to prepare the person to either battle the predator or flee. After the initial threat was encountered, the body's systems would return to normal.

But today, while we're less likely to run into a saber-toothed tiger on the commute to work, our bodies are still programmed the same way. Events that scare or worry or anger us produce this stress response, where breathing becomes faster and shallower, heart rate and blood pressure increase, and stress hormones like adrenaline and cortisol surge. The problem is that stress for many people becomes chronic, or constant, and that affects us both physically and emotionally.

I'll show you how to reduce stress in your day-to-day life. Beating daily stress can have a significant effect on your eating habits, too. Stress often compels people to skip meals, overeat, and/or eat lots of sugary, fatty foods. Also, researchers are finding that being subject to chronic stress affects hormones that make you more likely to gain weight around your middle and may make it harder to shed pounds.

That's one of the reasons I want you to do more than look at *what* you put into your body and do to your body. I want you to reflect on how you cope with stress. For example, I see a lot of people who are emotional eaters—they turn to food when they're angry, upset, lonely, depressed, or anxious. As a nutritionist I help them cope with their stress or with their other difficult feelings, and that helps with their eating as well. I'm not a psychologist, but sometimes emotional issues are what I call connecting points between nutrition, fitness, and wellness. You're overeating because you're stressed, and you rely on food to calm your nerves. When you learn how to manage your stress better, you also eat better—if you can cope with some of those underlying reasons, it frees you up to look at food a different way.

But the third part of my program is about more than managing stress. It's also about becoming more aware of your life, what makes you happy, and taking steps to enhance your happiness. Wellness is also about nurturing yourself and your relationships, because ultimately that's one of the keys to your health and happiness. Self-esteem and supportive, happy relationships contribute to health just as much as eating right and exercising. Maintaining good relationships—a sense of connectedness in your life—and having a sense of purpose all help you stay healthy, maintain your weight, and prevent disease just as exercise and eating well do.

Like the "Eating Well" and "Getting Fit" sections of my 12-Week Action Plan, small, specific action steps accompany each week for the "Feeling Good" component. However, while each of the twelve weeks' changes are critical to the "Eating Well" and "Getting Fit" elements, the core of the "Feeling Good" program is established once you reach the halfway point after the first six weeks. After that the "Feeling Good" action steps enhance the core plan but are less essential, so I have offered them as optional. I'd like you to try several of them, but I don't want you to feel overwhelmed by having to do them all. If you incorporate the "Feeling Good" action steps of the first six weeks, you'll have a solid, effective lifestyle plan in place. The changes in the weeks that follow are designed to further enrich your life. I suggest you try at least three of the "Feeling Good" changes in Weeks 7 through 12.

My plan has three elements—nutrition, fitness, and wellness—that are all interconnected. Becoming more emotionally healthy and reducing stress will make it easier for you to make smarter food choices and make you more likely to stick with your fitness routine. And when you work out regularly, you feel better about yourself and about your body, which helps with your overall happiness—and makes you more likely to want to eat better because you want to give your body the fuel it needs. Each element supports the others.

If you're unhappy with the shape of your body or the size of your thighs, it's natural to turn to a diet or exercise program in search of the results you want. But true fitness comes from integrating body, mind, and spirit. If you focus only on your external self, your life will feel empty. It's only by honoring your inner self and developing a healthy balance that you'll feel truly fulfilled.

how to use this book

This book is designed to walk you through small changes over the space of twelve weeks. But the way you use it is completely up to you. You can read through it all at once to get an overview of the program, and then follow it over the next three months—or you can start on a different week, depending on where you are and what your individual goals are. If you get sidetracked, you can always pick up where you left off, or use the chapters to brush up on ways to eat better, become more active, and live a healthier, less stressed, happier life.

The choice is yours. Ready to see how small changes add up to big results? Turn the page.

the 12-week action plan

After years of working and talking with hundreds of people who want to change their lives, I knew I wanted to design a simple, easy-to-follow program that provides the tools you need to change your life—in just three months. By making small changes every week—and building on those changes over time—you'll find that you can reach your nutrition, fitness, and lifestyle goals while you create new, healthier habits that will be easy to maintain in the future.

In these twelve weeks you will learn how to eat right for the rest of your life—and begin to do so. You will establish an effective, doable exercise regimen that you enjoy—and that you'll continue to enjoy in the future. You'll learn simple ways to reduce stress and increase your day-to-day happiness. And most important, you'll create a bridge between *knowing* what to do for good health and *doing* it.

BEFORE YOU BEGIN
get the lay of the land

Before you begin, I'm going to help you determine where you're at in terms of your diet, activity level, and lifestyle. Are you already eating well but unused to exercise? Do you work out regularly but still feel overwhelmed by stress? Or is your entire lifestyle in need of an overhaul? (If it is, don't worry—the 12-Week Action Plan will help you accomplish this.)

You may be tempted to skip this step—I can hear you already, "Come on, come on! I'm ready! Just tell me what to do!" But before you launch into the 12-Week Action Plan, take a few minutes to lay the groundwork. You'll have a sense of where you are, and get a better handle on what specifically you want to improve. And you'll have a solid "before" marker so when you've completed the plan you can see how far you've come.

To make this easy for you, I've developed a Lifestyle Questionnaire (page 21). Take this thirty-question quiz and then score your answers. You'll immediately have a clearer picture of what areas of your life need improvement—and a realistic idea of what you can accomplish in the next twelve weeks.

the food and exercise journal

Next, get a notebook and christen it your *Food and Exercise Journal*. This doesn't have to be anything fancy—a cheap, small memo book is fine. You just need a place to write down what you're eating and when, how much you exercised, how you felt afterward, and to keep track of the small changes you'll make over the next twelve weeks.

I know, I know—you're resistant to the idea. "I'm willing to do the program, but why do I have to *write* everything down?" may be going through your mind. Maybe you're thinking, Well, I'll just skip this step. I can do the program without the journal.

Let me explain why this journal is so important, and why I use it with clients. First of all, studies show that people who keep track of how much they eat have an easier time losing and maintaining their weight. Simply writing down what you consume and when makes you more aware of your caloric intake. But maintaining a food and fitness journal also becomes a motivational tool in itself. You'll be able to identify your eating and activity patterns, review your progress, and track your improvement in the weeks to come.

Still need convincing? Listen to the story of forty-year-old Jerry, a former client of mine. He came to me in a panic. His older brother had just had a heart attack. Fortunately, his brother had come through okay, but his father had died of heart disease in his late sixties. Jerry feared he was next. He was overweight and knew he had to make some changes in his diet, but he didn't know where to begin.

The first thing I had Jerry do was start a food journal. He wrote down *everything* he ate and drank, even if it was just a nibble or a sip. After a few days of journal keeping, one of Jerry's biggest challenges became crystal clear: Jerry was a nibbler. Every time he opened the refrigerator, he'd pop a piece of cheese into his mouth. When he walked by the front desk at his office, he'd grab a handful of candy from the bowl.

When we looked at his food journal together, Jerry was amazed. He couldn't believe how much all his nibbling could add up. When he stopped mindlessly munching all day long, he was on his way to lasting weight loss.

Jerry found the journal an invaluable tool. He was eating without thinking about it, but keeping the journal helped make him aware of his eating habits. Over time, he found that he could also use the journal to help him stay on track. Keeping the journal sometimes prevented him from overeating because he shuddered at the thought of writing down three or four doughnuts, or a sleeve of Oreos. He also enjoyed looking back to see how his eating had improved over time.

A few months and thirty pounds later, Jerry was able to keep track of his eating without keeping a daily journal. He had learned new, healthier eating habits. But even now, he sometimes relies on it as a maintenance tool, recording what he eats for a week or two when he feels he's getting off track.

Remember, the most important aspect of the journal isn't how big or fancy it is—it's using it every day. Choose something that's easy to carry, and slip it into your pocket or purse. That's all there is to it.

the "dear me" letter

Next, take a few minutes and write an important letter—to yourself. Write down all the reasons you want to make a positive change in your health. Is it to have more energy? To look and feel better? To be able to see your children grow up and have kids of their own? To live a more fulfilling, happier life? To look better in your jeans? (Hey, that's okay—a little vanity can be a good thing.)

Write what you want to accomplish, and why you want to make this positive change. Be as honest as possible—this letter is for your eyes only. After you've read the letter, keep it with you. If you feel your motivation flagging, take it out and reread it to remind you of why you're making this change. Regardless of what your spouse, friends, or children want for you, it's *you* who has to make the effort.

I believe that to make a change in your lifestyle, your must use your *head,* your *heart,* and your *hands.* Let me explain. You need knowledge about what to do (your head), you need the motivation to make the change (your heart), and you need the skills to enact the change (your hands). Your "Dear Me" letter is really the heart of the program—it reminds you of why you're doing this. When your life gets in the way—when you feel too tired to go for your twenty-minute walk or you're tempted to skip your healthy snack in favor of a handful of chocolate chip cookies—take out the letter and reread it. It can help keep you on track when you're tempted to stray.

asking for—and receiving—support

Another thing that can help keep you on track is the support of the people around you. The changes you make have an impact on your family, friends, and coworkers, and their response to your new behaviors can make a tremendous difference. Your

the numbers game

The Lifestyle Questionnaire and the "Dear Me" letter are both valuable tools, but there's sometimes no substitute for hard numbers. If you have "weigh-o-phobia" or tend to obsess over a number on the scale, you can skip this step. But if you're up to the challenge, weigh yourself before you start the program. If you hate the scale, simply measure your chest, waist, and hips with a tape measure—the numbers may surprise (or shock!) you, but remember they're only numbers. Like the Lifestyle Questionnaire, they'll give you a starting point, nothing more.

If, like many people, you like hard evidence to prove your progress, you've now got the figures you need. Make a note of them here—you'll compare the end results at the end of the twelve weeks. There is also a space at the end of each chapter to record your weight. Again, if you feel that regular weighing is not for you, feel free to skip this step. However, data from the National Weight Control Registry show that regular weighing in is one of the habits of people who have successfully lost weight and kept it off.

DATE _____

WEIGHT _____

CHEST (inches) _____

WAIST (inches) _____

HIPS (inches) _____

family will be affected when you stop keeping a lot of chips and cookies around the house and begin preparing different kinds of foods. Your coworkers will notice that you are going for walks during your lunch break instead of joining them at the greasy spoon. If the people in your life find your new behaviors threatening, or they don't understand why you are doing things differently, they may be discouraging or try to pressure you to go back to your old ways. So let everyone know you've decided to take better care of yourself, and tell them you need their help. Ask your family to keep an open mind to your new recipes and keep junk food out of your sight. Invite your coworkers to join you on your walks. With the backing of the people in your life, you'll be much more likely to succeed.

Another great way to get support is to ask someone to work this program with you. Has your neighbor said she'd like to lose some weight? Is one of your friends always talking about wanting to get in shape? Enlist them, and the two of you can help keep each other on track.

lifestyle questionnaire
how healthy are you?

Maybe you need to lose weight, but you're pretty good about balancing the demands of your daily life. Or maybe you already eat healthfully, but can't seem to find the motivation to exercise. Taking the Lifestyle Questionnaire will give you insight into how healthy your lifestyle is already—and what areas you can improve upon. (Don't forget to write down your score—you'll retake this at the end of the twelve weeks!)

As you answer, be honest with yourself. Don't select the answer that you'd *like* to say is true; choose the one that best fits your lifestyle now. Regardless of whether you score on the low side—or do better than you thought—you'll have a snapshot of your current habits to compare your progress to in the future.

NUTRITION CHECK

1. Do you agree with the following statement? "I'm usually aware of what and how much I'm eating."

    a. Yes—I try to pay attention to my food because I enjoy it more.

    b. It depends on how busy I am and whether I'm eating with my family.

    c. No—in fact, I often eat at my desk, in the car, or while watching television.

2. How often do you feel "stuffed" or overly full after eating?

    a. Rarely.

    b. Sometimes.

    c. Usually.

3. How often do you skip meals? (And no, coffee doesn't count as breakfast.)

    a. Rarely.

    b. Sometimes—it depends on my schedule.

    c. Frequently—I don't eat breakfast and lunch is often on the run.

4. **How much water do you consume on an average day?**
   a. Five glasses or more.
   b. Two to five glasses.
   c. Less than two glasses.

5. **How often do you snack on chips or other junk food? (Be honest.)**
   a. Rarely—and I pay attention to my portions.
   b. Sometimes.
   c. Frequently—I need my salt or sugar dose every day.

6. **What type of meats do you usually consume?**
   a. Skinless chicken breast, fish, or extra-lean cuts of beef or pork.
   b. Chicken with the skin, or trimmed beef or pork.
   c. Hamburgers, hot dogs, sausages, or marbled steaks.

7. **Your diet includes beans, nuts, and soy products like tofu:**
   a. frequently, if not daily.
   b. occasionally.
   c. rarely.

8. **How many servings of fruits and vegetables do you eat? (See page 238 for serving sizes.)**
   a. Five or more servings a day.
   b. Three or four servings a day.
   c. Less than two servings a day . . . and that's counting French fries.

9. **How many servings of dairy or other high-calcium foods do you consume every day? (See page 238 for serving sizes.)**
   a. Three or more.
   b. One or two.
   b. Less than one a day.

10. **You incorporate whole grains into your diet:**
    a. whenever possible.
    b. occasionally—you ask for whole wheat bread instead of white, for example.
    c. rarely.

11. How long can you walk fast without getting out of breath?

　a. Easily 30 minutes or more.

　b. For 5 to 10 minutes.

　c. Less than 5 minutes.

12. Think back to high school. How does your current weight compare with then?

　a. It's about the same.

　b. It's gone up about 10 pounds.

　c. It's gone up 15 pounds or more.

13. How active are you?

　a. Very active—I exercise 3 to 5 days a week, often vigorously.

　b. Somewhat active—I exercise 2 or 3 days a week, but I rarely break a sweat.

　c. Inactive—I don't exercise much at all.

14. How often do you stretch?

　a. Three times a week.

　b. Once a week, when I think of it.

　c. Never.

15. How often do you strength train or lift weights?

　a. Two or three times a week.

　b. Rarely—I don't want to bulk up.

　c. Never.

16. When was the last time you had fun during exercise?

　a. Within the last couple of days—I enjoy my usual routine.

　b. Recently, playing ball with the kids.

　c. I can't remember the last time I had fun exercising. It always feels like a chore to me.

17. When was the last time you tried a new physical activity, whether alone or with someone else?

    a. In the last month.

    b. In the last six months.

    c. I can't remember.

18. Your husband or partner has suggested a hiking trip this weekend. Your reaction?

    a. Great! It will be a chance to spend some fun time together.

    b. But I have so much to do—I can't afford the time.

    c. Absolutely not.

19. How often do you perform some form of sustained physical activity (like walking, gardening, or doing housework) for at least 20 minutes?

    a. Five times a week or more.

    b. Three or four times a week.

    c. Rarely—I'm too busy to exercise.

20. How satisfied are you with the overall state of your physical body?

    a. Pretty satisfied.

    b. I'd like to lose some weight and/or tone up.

    c. I'd like to have major reconstruction done.

WELLNESS CHECK

21. How easy is it for you to relax at the end of the day?

    a. It depends on the day. It is easy on most days.

    b. It's difficult—I feel like I have a never-ending to-do list.

    c. It's impossible. I couldn't relax even if I had the time.

22. How often do you eat to comfort yourself or relieve stress?

    a. Rarely.

    b. Sometimes.

    c. Often.

23. How often do you feel like you're living the life you want to?

a. Frequently.

b. Occasionally.

c. Almost never.

24. You'd describe your desk at work or home as:

a. fairly organized.

b. pretty disorganized, but I know where the important piles are.

c. mounds, mounds, and more mounds.

25. To you, the concept of mindfulness means:

a. living in the moment.

b. trying not to worry about the future.

c. trying not to hurt anyone's feelings.

26. How would you describe your sleep habits?

a. I usually feel rested when I wake up.

b. I could use extra sleep most mornings.

c. You need a forklift to get me out of bed.

27. How often do you feel emotionally out of control?

a. Rarely, unless I'm under extreme stress.

b. Occasionally.

c. Frequently.

28. How often do you take time to do something just for you?

a. Every day.

b. Occasionally.

c. Are you kidding? I've got a job and a family—I don't have time just for me!

29. How many close friends would you say you have?

a. Several.

b. One, but I can talk to her about anything.

c. I'm not that close to anyone.

30. When you think about the future, how do you feel?

   a. Excited—I have lots to look forward to.

   b. Worried that I'll never catch up on everything I have to do.

   c. I don't think about the future—it's too overwhelming.

Done? Now take a moment and add up your answers for each of the three sections. Give yourself 5 points for every **a,** 3 points for every **b,** and 1 point for every **c** answer, and write down your score:

NUTRITION SCORE: _____ (out of possible 50)

FITNESS SCORE: _____ (out of possible 50)

WELLNESS SCORE: _____ (out of possible 50)

TOTAL SCORE: _____ (out of possible 150)   DATE: _____

Take a look at your score, and consider the areas of your life that you'd like to improve. Now, if you've written your "Dear Me" letter and have designated a notebook as your *Food and Exercise Journal,* **you're ready to embark on the 12-Week Action Plan!** Come along. . . .

WEEK 1

THIS WEEK'S CHANGES:

1. **Shop for a healthy pantry.**

2. **Walk 3 times.**

3. **Practice a 5-minute breathing exercise daily.**

welcome to week 1! You may not realize it, but although you are just beginning, you've done a lot already. By picking up this book, buying it, actually *reading* it and getting to this point, you've moved from just thinking about changing your life to taking real action. Now let's keep the momentum going and dive into this week's changes.

EATING WELL
a healthy pantry

The first step toward eating well is having nutritious food at your fingertips. You can have the best intentions in the world, but if you have nothing good in your refrigerator, that's most likely what you'll wind up eating—nothing good. Sure, you can manage to eat right by relying on restaurants and takeout (see 6 Tips for Dining Out, page 29), but it's tough to do that every day. Studies show that people who often eat in restaurants have a much higher fat and calorie intake than those who prepare more meals at home. And it makes sense. When you cook your own meals you have the ultimate control over what you are eating. When you have healthy food on hand, you never have to worry about what you're going to eat next, and you're less likely to succumb to impulsive snacking and overeating. In short, having a stocked pantry takes the stress out of eating well and helps you stay on track.

You may be thinking you don't have time to shop for and prepare healthy meals. But you do—because I am going to help you make it easy and efficient. Once you invest a little time in stocking your pantry, you'll have everything you need to whip up a healthy meal faster than you can order a pizza. In this book I've given you dozens of quick, easy, and enticing recipes to try. You'll also have plenty of "eat-on-the-run" foods that you can grab as you head out the door. And in the end, you'll save money by forgoing all those restaurant and takeout meals.

First, look in your fridge, freezer, and cupboard and take inventory of what you

6 tips for dining out

1. PICK THE RIGHT RESTAURANT. While you can order healthfully in any restaurant, make it easy for yourself by choosing a place that has a reputation for serving healthfully prepared food. Restaurants specializing in seafood are usually a safe bet.

2. CHOOSE FOODS PREPARED WITH LESS FAT. Opt for foods that are steamed, poached, broiled, roasted, grilled, or baked. Avoid fried, battered, creamy, or cheesy choices.

3. MAKE SPECIAL REQUESTS. Don't be afraid to ask for sauces and dressings on the side, for food broiled without butter, or to say, "Hold the cheese." Most restaurants are happy to accommodate you.

4. KEEP PORTIONS HUMAN SIZED. Most restaurants serve ridiculously large portions. So try these ways to keep portions sensible:
- Eat just half your entrée and take the other half home.
- Order two appetizers instead of an appetizer and an entrée.
- Split your entrée with your dining partner.

5. START THE MEAL OFF ON THE RIGHT FOOT.
- If you can't eat just one or two slices of bread, ask the waiter not to bring the bread basket to the table.
- Start off with a garden salad, grilled vegetables, vegetable soup or consommé, or a shrimp cocktail to take the edge off your appetite.
- Skip the cream soups, fried vegetables, and cheese sticks.

6. DESERT DESSERT. Are you in the habit of having dessert after every meal? Break it and do the unthinkable: say "no thanks" to dessert. Or try a healthier choice like sorbet or fresh fruit.

have. Toss any frozen "mystery meat" and canned foods that have been in your home since you moved in—you know, the things like canned pumpkin that you never got around to using for Thanksgiving six years ago. (See the Storage Guidelines sidebar on page 32.)

Then, using the Healthy Shopping List below as a guide, make note of what you need and head out to the store.

healthy shopping list

Fresh Vegetables
Lettuce
Tomatoes
Cucumbers
Carrots
Celery
Avocado
Radishes
Mushrooms
Bell peppers
Broccoli
Spinach
Kale
Collard greens
Chard
Cabbage
Cauliflower
Eggplant
Zucchini
Green beans
Winter squash
Potatoes
Sweet potatoes
Corn
Onions
Garlic
Leeks
Scallions
Parsley
Cilantro
Rosemary
Basil
Tomato juice
Carrot juice
Other_____

Dried
Dried beans
Dried lentils
Split peas
Walnuts
Almonds
Pecans
Pine nuts
Peanut butter
Raisins
Apricots
Cranberries
Other_____

Soy
Soy milk
Tofu
Edamame
Other_____

Spices
Basil
Oregano
Cayenne pepper
Crushed red pepper
Cumin
Chili powder
Thyme
Sage
Cinnamon
Ginger
Bay leaves
Salt
Black pepper
Other_____

Fresh Fruit
Strawberries
Blueberries
Raspberries
Blackberries
Cherries
Peaches
Plums
Nectarines
Oranges
Grapefruit
Tangerines
Limes
Lemons
Pineapple
Honeydew
Cantaloupe
Watermelon
Grapes

Kiwi
Apples
Bananas
Pears
Orange juice
Grapefruit juice
Apple cider
Other_____

Dairy
1% or skim milk
Low-fat buttermilk
Low-fat or nonfat
  yogurt
Low-fat or nonfat
  cottage cheese
Part-skim
  mozzarella
Feta cheese
Reduced-fat
  cheddar
Parmesan cheese
Other_____

Oils and Condiments
Olive oil
Canola oil
Peanut oil
Sesame oil
Walnut oil
Cooking spray
Balsamic vinegar
Red wine vinegar
White wine vinegar
Cider vinegar
Mustard
Ketchup
All-fruit preserves
Low-sodium soy
  sauce
Low-fat mayonnaise
Olives
Cocoa powder
Brown sugar
Maple syrup
Molasses

Honey
Red wine
White wine
Dry sherry
Other_____

Grains
Whole wheat bread
Whole wheat pita
Whole-grain dinner
  rolls
Oatmeal
Whole-grain cold
  cereal
Whole-grain
  crackers
Baked tortilla
  chips
Corn tortillas
Brown rice
Wild rice
Pasta
Couscous
Bulgur
Quinoa
Whole wheat flour
All-purpose flour
Cornmeal
Baking powder
Baking soda
Other_____

**Fresh Meats,
Poultry, Fish**
Fish
Shrimp
Chicken breast,
  skinless
Turkey breast,
  skinless
Ground turkey,
  extra lean
Low-fat poultry
  sausage
Ham, extra lean
Beef, extra lean

Pork tenderloin, loin	Black beans	Applesauce	Broccoli
Venison	Garbanzo beans	Low-sodium soups	Peas
Ostrich	Low-sodium	Tuna in water	Vegetable medley
Eggs	chicken broth	Sardines	Stir-fry medley
Egg substitute	Crushed tomatoes	Salmon	Winter squash
Other_____	Diced tomatoes	Other_____	Veggie burgers
	Pasta sauce		Low-fat, whole-
Canned/Jarred	(low-fat)	**Frozen**	grain waffles
White beans	Pineapple (in juice)	Spinach	Other_____
Kidney beans		Corn	

Keep in mind that the Healthy Shopping List is quite extensive—it contains all the ingredients you'll need to make any recipe in this book. That doesn't mean you must buy everything on this list! You may want to look at the recipes peppered throughout the book and purchase the ingredients for the ones you want to try most. Ultimately, pick and choose what *you* like (and what your family likes) and get an appropriate amount for you and your family. Approach this initial shopping as the time to stock up on nonperishables. Buying bulk quantities of rice; cereals; and canned, frozen, and dried foods will free you to do just a light weekly shopping for the next month or so, and will save you money.

After your initial "stock-up" shopping trip, pick a convenient day and time to do your weekly shopping hereafter, and stick to it. If your schedule is flexible, you might ask the supermarket manager when the store receives fresh produce, and plan to shop on one of those days—you'll have a nicer selection to choose from. I recommend that each week you buy ingredients for salad (prewashed greens are a real time saver), four or five other fresh vegetables, and four or five different fresh fruits, depending on what looks most appealing and what's in season. That will get you in the habit of eating more fruits and vegetables and introduce you to new ones.

Also, if you eat on the go a lot, buy individual servings of foods like yogurt, cottage cheese, tuna, and applesauce so you'll have them handy. Having a stash of nuts and "portable" fruit like bananas, apples, and grapes also makes it easy to grab some healthy snacks on your way out the door.

The foods on this shopping list may look familiar from my "Usually," "Sometimes," and "Rarely" lists on pages 233–236. You'll notice that the Healthy Shopping List contains nearly all of the "Usually" foods, and a few "Sometimes" foods. So, while the only change you need to make this week is to establish a healthy pantry, I have an ulterior motive. And that is to get you to start eating those wonderful foods I recommend for an ideal diet.

Take a look in your cupboard again. How many of the foods there are on the "Rarely" list? If your house is loaded with "Rarely" items and you feel they will distract you from your new, healthier foods, consider giving away those foods to a neighbor or throwing them out. You don't have to get rid of them if you don't want to, but at least store them out of sight so your new and improved pantry takes center stage.

storage guidelines

FOOD	STORAGE FOR PEAK QUALITY
CANNED FOODS	
High-acid foods (tomatoes, pineapple)	12–18 months
Low-acid foods (most vegetables, meats, poultry, fish)	2–5 years
FROZEN FOODS	
Sausage, hot dogs, luncheon meat	1–2 months
Ground meat and poultry, stew meat, uncooked	3–4 months
Steaks, roasts, and chops, uncooked	4–12 months
Poultry, uncooked	9–12 months
Fish, uncooked	3–6 months
Cooked leftovers	2–6 months
Frozen dinners and entrées	3–4 months
PACKAGED/DRIED FOODS	
Pasta, rice (in airtight container)	1 year
Cereal, opened	2–3 months
Cereal, unopened	6–12 months
Peanut butter, unopened	6–9 months
Dried beans	1 year

recipes: rush-hour dinners

Most of the recipes in this book are quick and easy, but these three are super-express meals that take less than 15 minutes to make.

cuban-style black beans SERVES 6

These beans make a hearty main dish when served over rice. A salad of sliced tomato, avocado, and red onion is a perfect accompaniment.

2 15$\frac{1}{2}$-ounce cans of black beans

1 tablespoon olive oil

1 medium onion, diced (about 1 cup)

1 green bell pepper, diced (about 1 cup)

2 garlic cloves, minced

$\frac{1}{4}$ teaspoon dried oregano

1 teaspoon cumin

3 tablespoons cider vinegar

$\frac{1}{4}$ cup dry sherry or white wine

Drain the beans, put them in a colander, and rinse gently under cold water.

Heat the oil in a medium saucepan over a medium flame, add the onion, and cook for 3 minutes. Add the peppers and cook 3 minutes more, stirring occasionally. Add the garlic and cook for 1 minute. Stir in the beans, oregano, cumin, vinegar, sherry, and $\frac{1}{2}$ cup of water. Simmer on low for 5 minutes.

Calories 144; Fat 2.4 g (Sat .3 g, Mono 1.6 g, Poly 2 g); Protein 7.1 g; Carb 27.4 g; Fiber 8.7 g; Chol 0 mg; Sodium 622 mg

lemon-pepper chicken SERVES 4

Mark Bittman, cookbook author and *New York Times* columnist, showed me a version of this simple and delicious recipe when he was a guest on my TV show *Living Better*. It has been a rush-hour staple in my house ever since.

1 to 1$\frac{1}{2}$ pounds boneless chicken breast, pounded to a uniform $\frac{1}{2}$-inch thickness

$\frac{1}{2}$ teaspoon coarse salt

1 teaspoon freshly ground black pepper

2 teaspoons olive oil

$\frac{1}{4}$ cup freshly squeezed lemon juice

Pat the chicken breasts dry and season both sides with the salt and pepper. Heat olive oil in a large nonstick skillet over a medium-high flame. Place the chicken in the pan and cook for 6 to 8 minutes, turning once. Turn off the heat and pour lemon juice over the chicken. Serve.

Calories 160; Fat 1.8 g (Sat .5 g, Mono .4 g, Poly .4 g); Protein 32.8 g; Carb 1.3 g; Fiber 1 g; Chol 82 mg; Sodium 333 mg

I always have frozen shrimp on hand to make easy, elegant meals instantly. This lemony pasta dish is one of my favorites.

³/₄ pound linguini	**¹/₃ cup freshly squeezed lemon juice**
2 tablespoons olive oil	**¹/₂ cup white wine**
2 garlic cloves, minced	**1 cup chopped fresh, flat-leaf parsley**
1 pound large shrimp, peeled and deveined	**Salt and freshly ground black pepper to taste**

Bring a large pot of water to a boil. Add the linguini and cook according to the directions on the box. Drain, reserving 1 cup of the cooking water.

Meanwhile, heat the olive oil in a large skillet over a medium-high flame. Add the garlic and sauté for 1 minute. Add the shrimp and cook for 3 to 4 minutes, until the shrimp turn pink. Remove the shrimp from the pan and set aside. Add the lemon juice, white wine, and the reserved cup water to the skillet. Let simmer until the liquid is reduced by about half. Return the shrimp to the pan and stir in the parsley.

Add the drained linguini to the shrimp mixture, tossing to combine. Season with salt and pepper to taste.

Calories 529; Fat 10.2 g (Sat 1.5 g, Mono 5.4 g, Poly 1.9 g); Protein 34.6 g; Carb 68 g; Fiber 2.7 g; Chol 172 mg; Sodium 184 mg

the power of the pen: **the food journal**

Once you've got your pantry whipped into shape, I want you to begin to record in your journal everything you eat and drink. As I explained in "The 12-Week Action Plan," this is an amazingly effective, eye-opening exercise for most people. Many of us are accustomed to eating unconsciously, munching on whatever comes our way or tempts us at the moment. When it comes down to it, most of us have only a vague idea of how much we consume and our eating patterns. Writing down what you eat brings consciousness to your eating. It forces you to be aware of what and how much you eat and allows you to look back and see how you are doing.

Your journal should look something like this:

DATE:	Monday, March 8		
TIME	FOOD OR BEVERAGE CONSUMED	AMOUNT	NOTES
7:30	oatmeal	1 cup	satisfied after
	1% milk	1 cup	
	raisins	2 Tbs	

And so on. . . .

Write down when you ate, what foods you had, and the amounts (estimates are fine), and, if you'd like, how you felt afterward. I strongly recommend that you make your entries as they occur throughout the day, rather than filling it in each night, trying to remember what you had and when (you'll forget stuff, believe me!). Keeping the journal may seem like a nuisance at first, but stick to it—it will help you stay conscious of your eating and make you more aware of your usual habits.

ACTION

The first part of your action plan this week is to go shopping to revamp your pantry. The second component is simply keeping your food journal—writing down what you eat, when you eat, and how much. That's all there is to it.

GETTING FIT
the walking plan

Are you ready for the fitness part of the plan? If you're like many people, you're brimming with enthusiasm and good intentions. You're ready to get in shape, and you want results *fast*—like yesterday.

Slow down just a bit. When many people start exercising, they jump in head first. But overdoing it can lead to sore muscles, a sense of being overwhelmed, or even an injury. My plan will let you embark on your fitness plan at a safe, moderate pace that will prevent those aches and pains you may associate with exercise.

The object of this week is simple—to get you moving on a regular basis.

why walk?

It's so basic that we do it every day without thinking about it, but believe it or not, *walking* is the easiest way to get and stay fit. Even if you've never worked out before, you'll find it an efficient, effective method of exercise. And if you're an experienced exerciser, a regular walking routine may be easier to maintain than a more complicated program—you can walk practically anywhere with a minimum of equipment.

While you could use any form of aerobic exercise for the fitness component of my 12-Week Action Plan, I chose walking because of its universality. If you like, though, feel free to substitute another aerobic activity, such as biking, and follow the same workout program. The key is to enjoy what you're doing. So if walking is not for you, choose something you do like—you'll find it easier to stick with. Or mix it up by walking two days a week, and biking one day, if that makes it more fun.

Sometimes people find it hard to believe that simply walking can make such a big difference in the way they feel. But take Emma, a thirty-eight-year-old secretary at a law school. While Emma was committed to exercising regularly, with three school-age boys at home and a stressful job, the reality was that she found it nearly impossible to find the time to work out. She belonged to a local gym, but she was lucky to get there once a week. On top of that, the stress from work was taking a toll on her. She'd often find herself munching on the doughnuts and cookies that were always around the office to take the edge off during the day. Then at night, she'd have trouble unwinding and falling asleep.

Eventually Emma gave up the idea of going to the gym, and started walking during her lunch hour. Since she could eat lunch at her desk afterward, she was able to keep to a fairly regular walking schedule. And when she organized a lunchtime walking group with three of her coworkers, her fitness regimen really took off.

That was five years ago. Since then, Emma has lost ten pounds and kept them off, and says she's better able to cope with the demands of her job. Her group walks every day, Monday through Friday—indoors during the snowy Michigan winter and outdoors when the weather is good. "You won't cop out when someone else is depending on you," says Emma. "We encourage each other, push each other to walk a little faster, and the time goes faster." She says she doesn't even think about whether or not she is going to walk that day. It's automatic.

Besides giving her more energy and relieving stress, Emma says her walking eliminates her urge to eat junk food at work because she wants to hang on to the healthy feeling she gets from exercising regularly. She also finds it much easier to sleep at night. Emma believes her walking group has really made her life better, and she encourages people to find at least one person to walk with. "It makes it more regular, and more fun," she says.

finding the time

Emma faced one of the biggest reasons for not exercising—lack of time. That's one of the reasons I'm having you start off with a small time commitment—20 minutes 3 times a week.

But if you're wondering just when you're going to carve out even that small sliver of time, take a close look at your daily schedule. Can you walk first thing in the morning before your kids get up? During your lunch hour at work? While your daughter has piano lessons? Twenty minutes isn't a lot of time, and if you need to break it up into smaller chunks (say, two 10-minute sessions), that's fine, too.

One of the easiest ways to commit to an exercise program is to write it down in your calendar or date book, the way you would with any other appointment. After all, it's an appointment with yourself—and an investment in your overall health and fitness. At the beginning of the week, figure out when you'll put in your three sessions. Will you walk at lunch Monday, Wednesday, and Friday? Or get up early Tuesday and Thursday, and then walk around the soccer field during your son's game Saturday morning? Write down when you'll exercise and stick to it.

staying motivated

Some people find that the best way for them to keep to a regular regimen is to keep to the same route, covering the same blocks if they walk in town, or the same lanes or back roads if they walk in the suburbs or country. People who thrive on routine also try to find a regular time of day that is convenient, such as first thing in the morning or just before dinner, which helps them keep to a regular schedule. Very quickly, such regularity can allow you to "zone out," to think about other things as you walk, or to almost "meditate" as you exercise.

However, other people find such regularity and sameness incredibly boring. If this sounds like you, consider adding a number of variations to your triweekly walks. For example:

Walk in different locales The easiest solution to avoiding boredom as you walk is simply to take a different route. For example, walk through a park one day, along the river the next, or through a new neighborhood on the third day.

Many people enjoy walking in malls. This allows them to window-shop as they walk, and offers protection from the elements since most malls are covered. Some schools and colleges open their gym facilities to people in the neighborhood; walking on an indoor track at your local health club or YMCA is another option. Finally, if you have extra time on a weekend, drive to a park or other beautiful setting for a change of scene.

Find a walking partner Hook up with a buddy, and you're more likely to stick to your routine, and enjoy it more, too. Invite one of your friends who's always saying he or she needs to start exercising. Look around for potential walking partners—if you're a new mom, you might want to combine your walking regimen with that of another new mom, perhaps someone from your toddler's play group. You may even want to bring along the babies.

If you have teenage children, walking with them gives you an opportunity to catch up on their day. If you belong to a senior center or YMCA, post a sign seeking a fellow walker. Or encourage your spouse or partner to join you.

Not only does walking with a partner make the walk more fun, it tends to help you avoid procrastinating, keep up a vigorous pace, and stay on course with your regimen. Walking with a partner also allows you to maintain—and even stimulate—your social life as you exercise.

Walk the dog Most dogs need to be walked at least twice a day, so why not work your dog-walking duties into your walking regimen? Your pet will enjoy the exercise as much as you do, and benefit from it as well. Also, think about teaming up with another dog-owning neighbor, walking your dogs and "walking yourselves" at the same time.

Plan a destination One of the easiest ways to work a walking regimen into your life is to plan to walk to a destination such as your office, your kid's school, your own school, or your gym. If you live too far from your destination of choice, drive or take public transportation part of the way, then walk the remaining mile or so.

Use a treadmill Walking on a treadmill is one of the most effective ways to establish and maintain a walking routine. Treadmills are the most popular machines at health clubs and allow you to precisely monitor your pace, time, distance covered, and calories burned. They also enable you to walk at any time of day or night, no matter what the weather's like outside. Virtually all gyms have treadmills, or you can buy one and use it in the privacy of your home. (While having your own treadmill can make it easier to fit exercise into your schedule, quality treadmills are expensive. There are cheaper models available for several hundred dollars, but for a stable, safe machine, you'll probably spend at least a thousand dollars. You may want to hold off on purchasing such an expensive piece of equipment until you're sure it's worth the investment.)

one practical purchase

Since I'm discussing motivation, I'd like to share one of the best motivational techniques I know of: purchase a pedometer, a small device that clips onto your belt or waistband and measures the number of steps you take. At a cost of only fifteen to twenty-five dollars, it's an inexpensive tool that can help you track how much you're moving.

You may have heard the recommendation that people should take ten thousand steps a day to maintain good health. While that is ultimately a good number to shoot for, if you are relatively inactive, you might want to start with a more attainable goal and build from there. I suggest walking around with the pedometer for a few days and averaging your daily totals to find out your usual number of steps, then adding one thousand more as your goal. Once that becomes easy, add another thousand to your goal, and so on.

A pedometer gives you concrete evidence that you are meeting your goals, and gives you an incentive to take the stairs instead of the elevator. It's a fun way to track your walks and the rest of your daily activity, and you may be surprised by how much—or how little—you're already moving.

You can pick up a pedometer at any sporting-goods store. Some higher-tech models (from thirty to fifty dollars) include functions that tell you how far you've traveled and how many calories you've burned. But all you really need is a simple step-counter. It should be worn at your waist and centered at the midline of your right or left thigh (where the crease in your pants would be). Reset it to zero at the beginning of your day or walk, and you'll have a simple way of tracking your activity.

While you needn't have one to do the 12-Week Action Plan, I've found that clients who use them find them extremely motivating. Why not give it a try?

considering weather

If you have established your walking regimen in a gym, an indoor mall, or on a treadmill, you need not worry about the season or the weather. You'll be able to keep up your program whether it's the dog days of summer or the dead of winter. How-

keeping your cool in hot weather

These five tips will help you stay cool in hot weather. Keep in mind, though, that if the temperature or humidity (or both) is high, you may want to consider postponing your walk until the next day or walking in an air-conditioned gym or mall.

1. WALK DURING THE COOLEST HOURS OF THE DAY. Early in the morning is usually best in most locales, but if you live near a beach or lake, off-the-water breezes may cool the air in late afternoon. Avoid walking at midday, when temperatures usually peak.

2. AVOID DIRECT SUNLIGHT. Walk on the shady side of the street or along tree-lined hiking paths. If you walk where there's no shade, do it early in the morning or during early-evening hours, when it's cooler out.

3. COVER YOURSELF. Wear a baseball cap, tennis visor, or hat to shade your face. Wear sunscreen to protect your skin along with sunglasses and light-colored, lightweight clothing.

4. DRINK LOTS OF WATER. Before you start your walk, down a large glass of water. If you walk more than 30 minutes, carry a water bottle or stop for another drink during your walk. When you finish, drink another glass of water or two (at least a pint) to keep your body hydrated. Even if you don't notice yourself sweating, you *are* losing moisture; you don't need a soaked shirt to get dehydrated.

5. BEWARE OF HEAT SICKNESS. If you feel dizzy, nauseated, short of breath, chilly, or otherwise unwell, stop immediately, sit down, and drink some water. Don't be afraid to ask someone for help, or to help you get home. If you suffer from heart disease, diabetes, or any other medical condition, check with your doctor before walking in hot weather.

dressing warm in cold weather

If you don't like to exercise in the heat, cooler weather can be a blessing. Many people find it invigorating to walk outdoors, even if it is snowing. The key to staying comfortable is dressing in layers, which allow you to peel them off as you warm up during your walk.

1. START WITH THE BOTTOM LAYER. Choose underwear made from fabric such as polypropylene, Thinsulate, or silk, which draws sweat away from your skin.

2. ADD ON MORE. Include an insulating layer, such as fleece, pile, or down; add another layer if weather dictates; and finish with a comfortable water-resistant jacket. If the temperature permits, tights may be sufficient; if it's very cold, wear tights or long underwear under water-resistant pants or sweat pants.

3. HEADGEAR AND ACCESSORIES. In cold weather, wear a warm hat or ear band to protect your ears; a scarf will keep your neck warm. Slip on gloves or mittens—in particularly cold weather, gloves worn inside a pair of mittens will keep your fingers toasty. Waterproof walking shoes or hiking boots with heavy socks made of fabric that will wick perspiration will keep your feet warm. You may also want to take along lip balm, sunscreen, sunglasses, and a bottle of water—even in the cold, you can still get sunburned or dehydrated.

ever, if your regimen involves walking outside, you'll want to take the season—and the weather—into account.

Don't let this stop you, though—I encourage people to walk outside whenever possible. Outside, you can feel the sun on your face, smell fresh air, hear the sounds of birds, and enjoy your surroundings in a way that isn't possible indoors. Simply being outside can lift your spirits—research shows that people who walk *outside* feel happier and report a more elevated mood than people who walk the same distance indoors.

ready, set, walk!

At the beginning of your walk, start off slowly. Your muscles and ligaments aren't warmed up yet, especially if you walk early in the morning. After about 3 to 5 minutes, you can speed up so that you're walking at a comfortable pace. Your mission isn't to overexert yourself, but instead to get your body used to continuous exercise for 20 minutes. Slow your pace for the last several minutes of your walk—this is called the cool-down. When you finish, drink at least 8 to 16 ounces of water to replenish your fluid.

This week, you'll walk 3 times. This is frequent enough so that exercise will begin to be a habit. But it also gives your body (which may be unused to working out) a chance to adapt while minimizing soreness.

walk right, walk tall

You've been doing it since you were a baby, and chances are you probably don't think about the way you walk. But when you're walking for exercise, form becomes more important. When you walk, your head should be up, your chest lifted, and your legs centered under your hips. Your steps should be comfortable, and your arms should swing naturally as you stride along. You should be walking heel, toe, heel, toe—in other words, your heel should strike the ground first, then you roll onto the ball of your foot, and push off with each step.

If you tend to slump when you stand or walk, imagine a string attached to the crown of your head, pulling your body into alignment. Even hunching over a little will make you more prone to injury over the long haul. Proper form helps prevent this. When you walk, occasionally check your form. Your body shouldn't be ramrod straight, but you should maintain good posture throughout your walk.

the walker's closet: dress the part

One of the great things about walking is that you need a minimum of equipment to be able to do it. One item you shouldn't skimp on, though, is a good pair of walking shoes.

Shoes Walking shoes are designed to support your feet and minimize jarring, and they're well worth the investment. Look for shoes that fit comfortably, leaving a half inch or so in the toe box between the end of your foot and the shoe itself. They shouldn't pinch your heels nor be so loose that your foot moves freely as you step. If you have high arches, you'll want to select a shoe designed for your type of foot.

Your best option is to buy a new pair of shoes at a specialty shoe shop or a fitness store. You may spend a little more than grabbing a pair at your local superstore, but you're also more likely to get a pair of shoes that fit your type of foot. Your salesperson may want to look at your feet and the wear patterns of the shoes you're wearing to determine what type of shoe will be best for you. He or she may also ask how often you walk and on what surfaces, and what distances.

Socks Comfortable socks help support and cushion your feet while you walk. You can walk in any type of socks, but if you tend to get blisters, you may want to try synthetic fabrics over cotton. Socks with CoolMax, Supplex, or other synthetic blends are designed to draw sweat away from your skin so your feet feel drier and more comfortable. Thin socks may also reduce your chance of blisters—thick socks can bunch up and rub while you're walking.

Walking clothing Again, you can walk in just about anything. But clothing that doesn't restrict your movement is the best bet. You may be most comfortable in shorts, sweats, or tights on the bottom and a T-shirt or sweatshirt on top. If you're walking in cooler weather, dress in layers; then you can remove them as you warm up. If it's cold out, add a hat and gloves to your outfit; you'll warm up as you get moving, but you don't want to be chilled if you're walking outside.

for women only

You may want to consider one final addition to your walker's wardrobe: a decent sports bra. While walking is a lower-impact activity than jogging, unless you're small breasted, an athletic bra will help make your walks more enjoyable. (You don't want to worry about your chest bouncing around all over the place, and it's uncomfortable as well!)

There are two basic types of sports bras: compression bras and encapsulation bras. The former flatten your breasts against your chest, while encapsulation bras are designed to hold each breast separately. Try on a few to see which feels the most comfortable—if you're larger than a B cup, you'll probably want an encapsulation bra, which provides more support. Make sure that the seams don't rub or chafe; washing the bra before wearing it will make it softer.

gearing up

Now that you've got on appropriate workout gear, you're all set. I already discussed the benefits of using a pedometer, but if you're walking outdoors, you may want to add a few accessories:

Safety and reflective gear If you walk early in the morning or at the end of the day, reflective gear can save your life. You can find hats, gloves, vests, and other articles of clothing that have reflective surfaces as well as flashing lights and other attention-getting equipment that you can strap on your arm or your waistband. Wearing light-colored clothing, especially at dawn and dusk, makes you more visible to drivers, bicyclists, and others.

Carriers/fanny packs Want a place to stash your car keys, a small towel, a bottle of water, or a Walkman? Grab a carrier or fanny pack, strap it around your waist, and you're ready to go. Make sure that whatever you choose is comfortable and doesn't chafe or irritate your skin; it should fit snugly enough that it doesn't bounce a lot but not so close that it feels tight.

Water bottles For a 20-minute walk, you don't necessarily need to take water along. But for longer walks—or if you're exercising in hot weather—consider taking H_2O with you. An inexpensive plastic bottle with a snap-off or squirt cap will help you stay hydrated; some come with straps to make them easier to carry in your hand, while many will fit into a waist carrier designed to hold them.

Key holders If you like to travel light, you can buy a small key holder that straps onto your waistband or onto the laces of your walking shoes.

to tune in—or not?

Listening to music while you exercise is a great way to stay motivated—in fact, studies show that people can work out longer and at a higher level when they're "tuned in." Headsets are popular with walkers of all ages, and there are dozens of different kinds of cassette players, CD players, radios, and MP3 players you can buy; look for ones that are designed to be used during sports or fitness use.

A word of caution, though: if you wear a headset, be sure to keep the volume down low enough that you can hear what's happening around you. And be smart. While it's great to lose yourself in your music, don't wear them while walking in high-traffic or crowded areas where you need to pay attention to vehicles.

staying safe

If you walk at a health club or indoors, you may be less concerned with safety. But if you're walking outside, a few tips will help keep you healthy and safe. While anyone can be attacked while walking, women are particularly vulnerable, so take precautions:

1. WALK DEFENSIVELY. When you're outside, pay attention to your environment and who's around you. Walk with your head up and look at people as they approach you. Don't walk alone in isolated areas.

2. LOOK FOR CARS. The average driver is not looking for you—you're much smaller than another vehicle. Stay off the roads whenever possible, and choose routes away from heavily trafficked areas. Your mom taught you years ago to look both ways before crossing the street, but make sure you do, even at a stop sign—many drivers don't bother to stop completely and may not see you. If there's no sidewalk and you must walk in the street, walk facing traffic as far over on the shoulder as you can get. You're much safer facing traffic than walking with it.

3. WALK IN WELL-TRAVELED PLACES whenever possible—there's safety in numbers. Know where the nearest house or pay phone is, or carry a cell phone with you in case of an emergency. If you must walk alone after dark, stick close to your home or walk in a place that's relatively busy. (For example, a park near my home has baseball and soccer fields that are lighted during summer nights, and many people stroll the fields after dark.)

4. DON'T CARRY YOUR VALUABLES. Lock your purse or your wallet in your car, or leave it at home. Don't carry loads of cash or wear expensive jewelry, especially if you're walking in busy urban areas—you'll make yourself a target.

5. TELL SOMEONE WHERE YOU'RE GOING when you set out for a walk, and let them know when to expect you back. If you're walking in a new locale or park, take a map.

Walk for 20 minutes 3 times this week at any pace you'd like. When you have finished each walk, record your progress in your journal.

FEELING GOOD
better breathing

From the moment we take our first inhalation, we do it twenty-four hours a day, seven days a week, almost always without stopping to think about it. When you breathe, you deliver oxygen to all of your body's cells, including those in your brain. (If you've ever held your breath too long, and became light-headed, it's because your brain is being starved of oxygen.)

Normal breathing involves deep, slow inhalations and exhalations. When you're stressed, however, you tend to take shorter, shallower breaths, which don't supply as much oxygen to your body; this increases the amount of stress you experience. Breathing is fundamentally linked to the way we feel both mentally and physically—as a result, simply changing the way you breathe will enable you to handle stress better.

Sounds too good to be true? When I talk to people about the importance of proper breathing, I get a lot of skeptical looks. Yet deep, slow, focused breathing can change the way you feel, give you an emotional lift, and reduce stress and anxiety. Once you get in the habit of checking your breathing, you'll find that you can focus and center yourself simply by concentrating on the way you're inhaling and exhaling.

the 5-minute breather

You probably can't remember the last time you sat quietly and simply focused on your breath. This 5-minute exercise allows you to become aware of your breath, and slows down your heart rate and reduces your stress levels in the process. It's simple: just sit and be aware of your breathing. Inhale, exhale, and repeat. Your breath may begin to slow and deepen, but don't actively try to change it. Just follow it without judgment. How do you feel? How does paying attention to your breath change how you feel? How does it change your breathing? You may be surprised how relaxing this small step can be.

ACTION

Your action plan this week is simple: practice the 5-minute breathing exercise once a day. That's it!

WEEK 1
action summary

EATING WELL
- Stock your pantry with healthy foods.
- Write down what you eat, and when, in your journal.

GETTING FIT
- Walk for 20 minutes 3 times.
- Note your walks in your journal.

FEELING GOOD
- Do the 5-minute breather.

WEIGHT _____

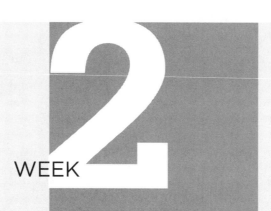

WEEK **2**

THIS WEEK'S CHANGES:

1. **Learn to identify—intuitively— when you are truly hungry, and stop yourself from overeating.**

2. **Get your 3-times-a-week walking program "up to speed."**

3. **Consider the concept of mindfulness, and begin to be mindful in all aspects of your life.**

EATING WELL

understanding hunger

I once asked a friend if she was hungry, and she answered, "What time is it?" Her reply was more profound than she realized, because it had nothing to do with actual hunger. She, like many people, had trained herself to disregard her true hunger, and instead relied on the clock to tell her when to eat.

By tuning out real feelings of physical hunger, we shut out one of our body's most basic messages, a signal to satisfy a fundamental need. By denying true hunger, we also open ourselves up to ignoring the other side of the hunger—satiety, or the sense of feeling full. Once we start eating, we often don't know when to stop, and as a result lose one of our most basic weight-management tools.

People overeat all the time simply because the food is there, because it is a good value to buy the "larger" item, or because a dining partner is still eating. Whatever the reason, the underlying problem is that we are ignoring our body's signal that it has had enough.

eating like a baby

We all come with a built-in hunger-satiety system. Just watch the way a baby eats to see how well it works. When infants are hungry, they demand food and eat enthusiastically. They may pause to rest awhile, eat some more, then gradually they stop. You cannot force-feed infants. When they have had enough, they simply stop.

As we get older, this connection with our true hunger and satiety is often drowned out by other food cues we are bombarded with every day. As children, we got gold stars for "cleaning our plates," and we learned to associate hamburgers, hot dogs, chips, ice cream, cake, and candy—all of which are filled with fat, sugar, and/or additives and preservatives—with carefree summer picnics, birthday parties, and other happy occasions. Food companies throughout the world spend millions every year to make our mouths water in advertisements for such items as finger-lickin' chicken, double-crust pizzas, and sugar-laden sodas. After we've been seduced by these cultural signals and have gained too much weight, we go on highly restrictive diets, which only cause us to get further out of touch with our true feelings of physical hunger and satiety. And on it goes.

The good news is you can get back to that fundamental, babylike place of eating intuitively. When you do, you will not only have the fuel you need to be energized throughout the day, but you will also be healthier—and, if need be, thinner.

eating intuitively

Take a look at the Hunger Continuum, below. It represents the relative degrees of hunger, starting with 1, for "Famished/Starving," something few of us ever experience, and progressing through 10 for "Painfully Stuffed," which is the sensation of being so full of food that we might actually feel ill. The goal is to stay in the center of this scale, between 3 and 6, throughout the day. To do this you have to listen to your body—to identify when you are truly, physically hungry. Not bored hungry, lonely hungry, or stressed-out hungry, but truly, stomach-growling hungry. And you have to know when you are satisfied. It takes some practice, but once you tap into these cues you will have discovered the most natural form of portion control.

Ideally, you want to eat only when you are truly hungry. If you find yourself reaching for food for reasons besides true hunger, ask yourself why. It may be because you have a designated lunch hour and need to eat at that time, or because you are making an effort to eat breakfast. That is fine. It is not always logistically possible to eat according to your hunger, and it *is* a good idea to maintain a basic eating schedule, including breakfast. (I'll get more into that next week.) But beyond that, try not to eat unless you are physically hungry. And don't start eating when you get your first little hunger signals—a bit of hunger is good. It means your body is starting to tap into your fat stores for energy. When your hunger is stronger, but not overwhelming, say at level 3, your body's cues should not be ignored. Then it is time to eat.

hunger continuum

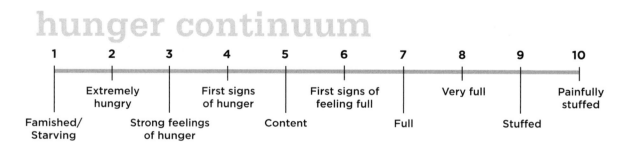

knowing when to stop eating

The opposite end of the spectrum of knowing when you feel physically hungry is knowing when to stop eating. It is important to quit when you are "content," at about number 5 on the Hunger Continuum. All of us have had the experience of eating a delicious meal and reaching a point where we say to ourselves, "I could stop now," but the food is so good that we keep on eating. That is *precisely* the point where we must stop. Most of us are so used to eating way beyond the satiety point that stopping may feel odd at first. However, remind yourself that 20 minutes after you stop eating, once your stomach sensors have had time to tell your brain you are satisfied, you will feel content and energized, not sleepy and sluggish, the way you feel after you have overeaten.

The key to recognizing this seemingly magical satiety point is to eat slowly, chew each bite, and stop periodically to check in with yourself and note how you are feeling. Slowing down, in particular, works wonders. You will find that you not only eat less, you will enjoy your food more. (You don't really taste your food if you are

five ways to feel full faster and eat less

1. USE A SMALL PLATE. As the saying goes, "We eat with our eyes." With a smaller plate, you can trick your eyes into thinking your portion is bigger than it is.

2. FILL UP ON VEGETABLES. Foods that pack a lot of fiber and water, like vegetables, fill you up fast without a lot of calories.

3. START WITH SOUP. Studies show that people who start their meal with a broth-based soup, especially a chunky soup, eat less at the following meal, and fewer total calories throughout the day.

4. DON'T HEAP THE FOOD ON YOUR PLATE. The more you put in front of you, the more you'll eat. Instead, take a small amount and go back for seconds after waiting 10 minutes, if you are not yet satisfied.

5. BUY THE "SMALL." Research shows that people eat more when they are given a bigger package of food. So always get the smallest size package available.

shoveling it in.) Best of all, your digestion—and your overall health—will improve.

Once you tap into eating intuitively and respond to your hunger-satiety cues, you will find it easier to leave food on your plate. You will also see that portion control doesn't have to be a painstaking chore; instead, you will discover that it really is innate for each of us—if you are only willing to listen to your body.

is your hunger physical or emotional?

Another reason some of us have problems determining true physical hunger is that we confuse physical hunger with "emotional hunger" or other feelings that we believe can be satisfied by eating. Deciding whether you are physically hungry or, in fact, emotionally hungry can be tricky and may require some concentration and awareness. But simply pausing for a moment before reaching for food and asking yourself the true nature of your hunger can help.

As a society, we have learned to eat for all sorts of reasons other than physical hunger. We eat "for joy," such as to celebrate an event, like a wedding, birthday, or holiday. We eat because we think we "deserve it" because we've had a rough day at work, we finally cleaned out the garage, or even because we walked a mile! We eat because we're sad, from a bit depressed to grieving. We eat because we've just met the love of our lives or we eat because we're lonely. We eat because we're stressed out, overworked, or overwhelmed, or we eat because we're bored or tired.

Unfortunately, emotional hunger is most often associated with negative feelings, such as anger, loneliness, frustration, and fear, and is frequently characterized by depression and hopelessness. If you find that you are reaching for food to satisfy these sorts of feelings, try talking with your spouse, calling a friend, or writing in your journal, to get at what's bothering you. If you experience emotional hunger frequently or are unable to curb it, consider going for professional help.

eating out of habit

Another kind of emotional hunger results from old habits, especially the pleasant ones that are associated with feelings of comfort and security. (Eating regular meals and snacks is also a habit, but it is a good one, as I'll explain next week.)

Remember when you used to come home from school and Mom would give you a glass of milk and couple of cookies? Maybe you weren't really hungry, but your mother was using food as a way to mark the end of the school day and to tide you over until dinner. And wasn't it nice? Didn't you feel loved and cared for?

Many of us have transmuted this kind of old, comforting gesture into a not-so-good adult habit. We use food as a way to separate one part of the day from another, or one activity from another. We're finished vacuuming, so we head for the refrigerator; we've walked for 20 minutes, so we reach in the cookie jar. The moment we arrive home from work, we have a drink or crackers. Most of the time, we aren't hungry; it's just a habit—and it feels good.

The first step to coping with emotional hunger is simply to be aware that you are not physically hungry but are using food to satisfy some other need. The next step is to substitute food with some other activity to deal more constructively with the feelings. For example, if you are eating out of stress, do the 5-minute breathing exercise, take a warm bath, or go for a brisk walk. If you're feeling sad or lonely, don't turn to ice cream—just call a friend, write a letter, or write in your journal. If you need a reward for working hard, get yourself a new CD instead of rewarding yourself with food.

recipe

minestrone soup SERVES 6

A cup of this chunky soup at the start of a meal just may be a perfect appetite appeaser. A bowl of it with some whole-grain bread and a salad makes a hearty meal.

2 tablespoons olive oil

1 large onion, diced

2 garlic cloves, minced

4 carrots, diced

2 stalks celery, diced

1/2 teaspoon dried basil

1/2 teaspoon dried oregano

28-ounce can of crushed tomatoes

48-ounce can of low-sodium chicken broth or vegetable broth

1 cup canned kidney beans, drained and rinsed

3/4 cup elbow macaroni

Salt and freshly ground black pepper to taste

Grated Parmesan cheese (optional)

Heat the oil in a large stockpot over a medium flame. Add the onion and cook until soft, about 5 minutes. Lower the heat to low-medium. Add the garlic, carrots, and celery and cook for about 10 minutes more, or until the vegetables are tender, stirring occasionally. Add a bit of water if the mixture gets too dry while cooking. Add the basil and oregano and stir to combine.

Add the tomatoes and chicken broth and bring to a boil. Lower the heat to low-medium, add the beans and macaroni, and let simmer for 15 minutes. Season with salt and pepper to taste. Garnish with a sprinkle of Parmesan cheese.

Calories 238; Fat 6.9 g (Sat 1.5 g, Mono 3.6 g, Poly .9 g); Protein 10.3 g; Carb 36.8 g; Fiber 7.8 g; Chol 3.8 mg; Sodium 455 mg

ACTION

Every time you eat something, register your level of hunger when you begin and your level of satiety when you finish, based on the Hunger Continuum, page 50. Note these levels in your journal. Try to stay between 3 and 6. ■ Also, if you'd like, record any feelings of emotional hunger in your journal. What are the feelings? Loneliness, anger, frustration, fear, boredom, fatigue? What did you do about the feelings? How often do you experience them?

GETTING FIT
walking with purpose

For Week 1, the object was quite simply to get you moving on a regular basis. Now that you've been walking regularly for one week, you are ready to take your regimen to a slightly higher level.

how hard should you exercise?

Last week you walked for 20 minutes at a comfortable pace at least 3 times—or you did enough shorter walks to meet this time requirement. How did you feel? You probably noticed that you felt less stressed afterward—or perhaps you were in a better mood. If you haven't exercised before, consider yourself introduced to regular workouts. Making the commitment and making the time—that's all there is to exercise.

Not all exercise is created equal, however. In general, the more challenging a workout feels, the more benefits you can reap from it. But that doesn't mean you have to suffer to be fit—so you can forget the old "no pain, no gain" theory. It's true that you can't just saunter along for 20 minutes 3 times a week and expect to radically change your health. You do need to push yourself a little bit to get fitter—what I call exercising along the edge, where you can feel that you're challenging yourself but you're not in agony or in pain.

When you're beginning an exercise program, however, you want to up the ante *gradually*. There are several ways to make a workout more challenging: you can do it for a longer period of time; you can exercise more frequently (say, five days a week instead of three); or you can increase the intensity at which you exercise.

In this chapter, we'll focus on the third element—intensity. With this program, you'll use three different levels of intensity:

- **Level 1: Low-Intensity Walking** is relatively slow, yet purposeful walking. This type of exercise helps to build stamina and cardiovascular strength, and serves as an excellent fitness walk for beginners. Low-intensity walkers average about 3 miles per hour and cover 1 mile in about 20 minutes. This is the level of walking we will focus on for the next few weeks of this program.
- **Level 2: Mid-Intensity Walking** is a brisker-paced walk where the walker typically moves at about 4 miles per hour, covering a mile in about 15 minutes. We will reach this level of walking at Week 6 of this program.
- **Level 3: High-Intensity Walking** is very fast walking that may include periods of jogging or running where walkers zip along at about 5 miles per hour, covering a mile in about 12 minutes. This form of walking is great for burning calories and shaping muscles. We will get to this level at Week 10.

For the next few weeks, you'll maintain the same basic workout plan of walking 3 days a week, for 20 minutes each time. To make the walk more challenging, you'll focus on its intensity, or how hard your body is working, and start to push yourself—you're going to begin to "walk harder."

finding the right intensity

Listen to Your Heart There are a number of ways to help determine the intensity of any workout. One of the most common is to use your heart rate to track how fast your heart is beating. The faster your heart beats, the harder your body is working. (You've probably seen people at the park or gym taking their pulse during or after exercise—they're measuring their heart rate.)

You may find it helpful to determine the range of heart rates that reflects the level at which you wish to work. This range is called your target heart-rate zone. Your target zone is based on your maximum heart rate, or "max," which is the fastest your heart can possibly beat. There are several different formulas used to calculate max;

see the box on page 57 to calculate your target heart-rate zone for each of the three walking levels.

Once you determine your target heart-rate zone, you simply measure your heart rate, or pulse, to ensure that you are walking at the right intensity. To measure your heart rate during exercise, slow down to a comfortable pace and place your index and middle fingers at the pulse point on your wrist or at the groove under the left side of your jaw on your neck. Count the number of beats you feel in 15 seconds and then multiply that number by 4 to get the number of beats per minute.

Another option is to purchase a heart-rate monitor. There are dozens on the market, and they are accurate and easy to use. You simply strap a monitor around your chest, and your heart rate is displayed continuously on a monitor you wear on your wrist. With higher-end models you can program in your training zones, and an alarm will go off if you begin working too hard (or cheat a little and slow down!).

bells and whistles: shopping for a monitor

If you're looking for a heart-rate monitor, don't be confused by the wide selection available. While there are dozens of models available, all fall into three basic types:

- Continuous read monitors—the simplest and least expensive; the monitor simply displays your heart rate. For many exercisers, this is all you'll need. (Price range, about sixty to a hundred dollars)

- Zone monitors—the most popular version. These allow you to program a training zone into the monitor; an alarm goes off if you stray from it. Different models have different features—some display both your heart rate and your percentage of max (so you don't have to calculate it); others include an automatic calorie counter as well. (Price range, about ninety to two hundred dollars)

- Downloadable monitors enable you to download your workout information onto your computer postworkout; they're great for serious athletes and techies. (Price range, about two to four hundred dollars)

Check out your sporting-goods store or order on-line at www.body tronics.com, www.heartmonitors.com, www.polarheartratemonitors.com, or www.cardiosport.com.

calculating your target heart-rate zone

There are several different methods used to calculate maximum heart rate, or max, but here's one of the most common:

Step 1. Calculate your maximum heart rate.

Your maximum heart rate is 220 minus your age. For example, if you are 40 years old, your maximum heart rate is 220 − 40 = 180 beats per minute

Step 2. Find your target heart-rate zone.

- For Level 1, low-intensity walking, the target heart-rate zone is 50 to 60 percent of your maximum heart rate. Multiply your maximum heart rate by .5 and .6 to find your low-intensity zone.
- For Level 2, mid-intensity walking, your target heart-rate zone is 60 to 70 percent of your maximum. Multiply your maximum heart rate by .6 and .7 to find your mid-intensity zone.
- For Level 3, high-intensity walking, your target heart-rate zone is 70 to 90 percent of your maximum. Multiply your maximum heart rate by .7 and .9 to find your high-intensity zone.

For example: for a 40-year-old walking at Level 1, low-intensity: 180 × .5 = 90 and 180 × .6 = 108.

The target heart-rate zone is 90 to 108 beats per minute.

Perceived exertion Measuring your heart rate is certainly a useful way to calculate the intensity of your exercise, but sometimes all those numbers can make your head spin! Personally, I like to use a scale called the Perceived Exertion Scale (see page 58), which is designed to estimate the intensity of exercise based on how you *feel* as you are working out. It correlates very well with the target heart-rate zone formula, so feel free to use either one—or both.

On the Perceived Exertion Scale, low-intensity walking corresponds to level 5 or 6, so walking should feel somewhat difficult. Mid-intensity walking corresponds to level 6 or 7, and should feel difficult, but not extremely so. And high-intensity walking corresponds to levels 7 to 9, so walking at high intensity should feel somewhere between difficult and extremely difficult.

Talk Test The talk test is another easy way to gauge exercise intensity. By talking aloud as you walk (or run), you can get a general idea of how hard you are working out. For low-intensity walking, you should be able to carry on a conversation with a walking partner, albeit a rather breathy one. Later, as you move to walks of greater intensity and duration, you may be able to speak only in snatches, or ultimately be able to get out only a word or two when you are working your hardest.

perceived exertion scale

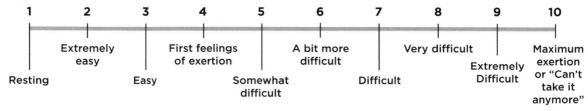

ACTION

Your goal this week is similar to last week's—to walk 20 minutes 3 times. But now begin to pay attention to your pace. Your walks should feel somewhat difficult, at Level 1, low-intensity. Also try speeding up your pace a few times to push yourself a little harder—you'll start to get a feel for what medium-intensity exercise is like.

FEELING GOOD
becoming mindful

At its most simplistic, mindfulness is being fully aware of your present moment. When you are being mindful, you are not judging or reflecting—you're not even really thinking. You are simply observing the moment in which you find yourself.

When you are being mindful, you have no other purpose than being awake and aware of that moment.

Mindfulness is both simple and complex. In Buddhist thought, it is an integral part of deep meditation, and takes years, even lifetimes, to fully understand. At the same time, it can be experienced, in a simple yet effective way, by anyone right at this moment.

This week you'll begin to experiment with mindfulness—just for a moment once a day. Instead of listening to the ever-present mental chatter most of us have ("I need

eating mindfully

I often have clients conduct a classic meditation exercise that involves slowly eating a raisin. I have them take *one* raisin and concentrate on the experience of eating it—from first enjoying its texture and aroma to gradually chewing and savoring the taste. When they stop to focus on this exercise, people are always amazed at how much flavor is contained in one tiny fruit.

One of the goals of the exercise is to teach you to slow down and really appreciate food and all its sensory properties. The frenzy of everyday life often leads us to gobble down our food mindlessly. But thoughtless, speedy eating isn't satisfying and can cause overeating and digestive problems. The next time you sit down to a meal, try these exercises, and encourage your family and friends to participate.

- **SAY GRACE.** Offering thanks—to God or whomever you wish to thank—not only for the delicious food but the abundance we enjoy, calms you and focuses your mind on this activity.

- **CONSIDER THE FOOD.** Instead of grabbing for your fork, enjoy the smell and look of the food before you begin to eat—what gourmets call the presentation.

- **EAT SLOWLY.** You don't need to chew each bite 40 times, but do savor each bite, chewing slowly. Experience the food's complex and subtle flavors.

- **PAY ATTENTION.** Even when you are eating on the go, find a moment to focus mindfully on your eating experience. You'll feel more satisfied if you concentrate on your food instead of trying to work, read, or watch television while you eat.

exercising mindfully

You can approach any activity in a mindful way, and that includes exercise. For example, as you're walking, don't try to think about all the things you have to do, or that you wish you were anywhere but on that treadmill or walking around that track. Instead of wishing the moment away, relish it. Get in touch with your body. Notice how your muscles feel, how your body is breathing deeply, and how good it feels to be moving. If you are outdoors, observe the trees, the sky, the water—whatever makes up your environment. Be in the moment.

to go to the store and get milk," "What should I make for dinner tonight?," "What's the stock market going to do next?," "I hope my job is safe with all the cutbacks lately," "This place is a pigsty!"), simply stop and focus on the present moment.

Check in with your physical body. How do you feel? Are you feeling energetic, alert, tense, anxious? Or tired, relaxed, sleepy, overwhelmed? What thoughts are racing through your head? Take a few minutes to sit and simply let yourself become aware of your surroundings and your body. A good time to do this might be toward the end of the afternoon at work, or while sitting in traffic, or even after dinner.

If you are having trouble quieting your mind, use the breathing technique you have been practicing for the past week. Traditionally, focusing on the breath, as you have been, has been used as a path to mindfulness.

Your mindful moment can be a good time for you to reflect and be thankful. It's easy to get distracted by the things that are "wrong" in our lives—jobs we don't enjoy, conflicts with our loved ones, financial pressures, worries about what's happening in the world today. But I find that stopping and simply focusing on a few things that I'm grateful for calms me and puts me in a more positive frame of mind. It could be something as simple as the fact that the sun is shining or my daughter is babbling happily to herself or I had a great night's sleep. Try counting your blessings the next time you feel overwhelmed or irritable—you'll be amazed at how much you have to be thankful about.

ACTION

Take at least one moment each day to stop and focus on the present moment, to be mindful.

action summary

EATING WELL
- Shop once this week to keep your pantry stocked with healthy foods.
- Stay between 3 and 6 on the Hunger Continuum and register your hunger and satiety level in your journal.
- Maintain your food journal.

GETTING FIT
- Walk for 20 minutes 3 times at Level I, low-intensity, or Level II, mid-intensity.
- Note your walks in your journal.

FEELING GOOD
- Do the 5-minute breather.
- Practice mindfulness at least once a day.

WEIGHT _____

THIS WEEK'S CHANGES:

1. **Eat three small meals and one or two snacks daily.**

2. **Add stretching to your walking regimen.**

3. **Learn how to manage your time according to your priorities.**

EATING WELL
the optimal eating pattern

For the past week you have been trying to eat more intuitively—eating when you are physically hungry and stopping when you are satisfied. You probably find you are eating smaller amounts than you did before, and you may be surprised to find how little it takes to make you feel full. Doesn't it feel good to not feel stuffed after dinner?

But as I mentioned in the last chapter, just as it is important to eat only when you are truly hungry, it is also important to have a basic eating schedule. This week you'll begin to guide your body into an optimal eating pattern—one that will keep you energized all day, help reduce cravings and impulsive eating, and may even help you lower your cholesterol.

The meal pattern that I find works best for most people is three meals and one or two snacks in regular intervals throughout the day. That may sound like a lot, but the key here is keeping those meals and snacks *small*. (See the Appendixes, page 240, for sample days with appropriate portion sizes.)

At first you may find that eating so frequently goes against your hunger cues. Many people tell me they are not hungry for breakfast, for example, or they prefer to skip lunch. But if that's the case, chances are you have trained your body into the all-too-common trap of eating little throughout the day and overeating at night. I have counseled dozens of people who regularly have nothing but coffee and some fruit or a bagel all day, only to eat a gargantuan dinner at night. Consuming most of your daily calories in the evening is bad for your digestion and it deprives your body of fuel when you most need it—during the day. It also sets you up to skip meals again the next day. After all, who is hungry for breakfast after sleeping on a big, heavy dinner?

When you start eating more throughout the day and less in the evening, you'll begin to wake up hungry, eager for breakfast. Your stomach will let you know when it's time for lunch. This catches a lot of people off guard. They feel uncomfortable with that hunger, which may be new to them, and fear it will make them eat more in the long run. But it won't. Research shows that people who skip breakfast usually wind up overeating later in the day, making up for the calories they tried to save, and then some. In fact, people who eat breakfast tend to be leaner than those who skip it. They also perform better on cognitive tests, and they are more likely to meet their nutrient needs overall.

One of the biggest benefits of adopting the three-meal/two-snack pattern is that it keeps your energy high throughout the day. Eating regularly helps stabilize your blood sugar, also known as glucose. When you go too long without eating, your blood sugar dips, and since glucose is the brain's primary fuel, those dips can leave you foggy, fatigued, irritable, and light-headed. You know that crabby, edgy feeling you get when you haven't had lunch and you're quick to snap at your kids or your coworkers? That feeling magically disappears when you eat at regular intervals. And as a bonus, research proves that people who eat more frequently have lower total cholesterol and more good cholesterol than people who skip meals!

Eating regularly also helps you eat healthier. Meal skippers are more likely to make impulsive—and usually unhealthy—food choices. It's a lot harder to resist

high-energy eating

If you experience energy slumps throughout the day, it may be your diet that's bringing you down. These energy-boosting tips can help get you back to speed.

- Don't skip meals or go more than five hours without eating. Skipping meals makes your blood sugar dip and deprives your brain of the fuel it needs to function optimally.

- Include some protein at each meal or snack. Protein-rich foods like fish, poultry, lean meat, eggs, beans, nuts, yogurt, milk, and cheese help prevent that sleepy feeling you can get after a meal; they also take longer to digest, so you feel full longer.

- Avoid sugary foods and refined starches like white bread. These foods can cause blood sugar to spike quickly and then fall again, causing energy lows.

- Avoid large, fatty meals. Large, heavy meals leave you feeling sluggish. It may be that your body has to work overtime to digest them.

- Drink plenty of water and other fluids. Fatigue is one of the first symptoms of dehydration, so drink plenty of water throughout the day to stay energized.

12 quick high-energy snacks

Going too long without eating can make you feel tired, cranky, and spacey. Small, healthy snacks or minimeals that include protein and carbohydrates will help keep your energy levels high throughout the day, and they take little time to prepare. Most of these make a good breakfast on the go, too.

1. Sliced apple with peanut butter (1 tablespoon)

2. Turkey (2 slices) and tomato on whole wheat bread (1 slice)

3. Low-fat cottage cheese ($1/2$ cup) and a peach or pear

4. A hard-boiled egg and a piece of fruit

5. Almonds ($1/3$ cup) and dried apricots ($1/4$ cup)

6. A yogurt-and-fruit smoothie (12 ounces) ($11/2$ cups)

7. Hummus ($1/4$ cup) and baby carrots (1 cup)

8. Low-fat yogurt (1 cup) and fresh strawberries (1 cup)

9. Baked sweet potato ($1/2$ potato) with low-fat cottage cheese ($1/2$ cup)

10. Baked tortilla chips (10) and low-fat bean dip ($1/2$ cup)

11. Reduced-fat cheese ($11/2$ ounces) and whole-grain crackers (5)

12. Half a peanut butter and banana sandwich (1 tablespoon peanut butter)

those M&M's on your coworker's desk when your head is spinning from not having eaten all morning. And when you have starved yourself all day, you somehow feel deserving of a few extra pieces of bread slathered with butter and a hunk of chocolate cake at dinner.

Having a set meal pattern also helps prevent that evening eating frenzy, where dinner has no real end but drags on from one snack to the next until you roll yourself into bed. With a set meal pattern, you stop eating for the day after dinner or a small evening snack. You may want to pick an absolute time to stop eating if nighttime nibbling is an issue for you.

As I said, the meal pattern I recommend is three moderate meals (breakfast, lunch, and dinner) and one or two small snacks a day, one mid-morning and one mid-afternoon. But that pattern isn't the only way to go. Some people prefer to graze, eating six smaller meals throughout the day. Others find it works better for their weekend schedule to eat two meals (brunch and dinner) and two or three snacks.

Whatever pattern you prefer, remember the mid-afternoon snack is key. Around three or four o'clock, most people's energy levels start to flag. That's when they reach for the chocolate and caffeine, and hope to summon the energy to exercise or get through the rest of their day. But if you plan to eat a healthy snack at that time, you'll be amazed at how much more stamina you have, how much more you can put into your walks, and how much easier it is to avoid overeating at dinner. You'll also be less likely to inhale whatever's in your refrigerator or pantry when you come home from work, and be willing to take the time to make a healthy dinner.

You may be thinking that you hardly have time to prepare and eat one healthy meal a day, much less three meals plus snacks. But it is not as difficult as it sounds. Look at the snacks on the previous page—neither they nor the meals have to be elaborate creations. And although it is important to sit down to a relaxed meal whenever possible, it is perfectly fine (and often necessary) to eat on the go. With the pantry you established in Week 1 and a little prep work, you have plenty of options that work in a time crunch.

healthy fast food

One typical fast-food meal can contain a full day's worth of fat and calories. But you can make the most of the drive-through by making smarter choices. Next time you are grabbing some fast food, get one of these healthier options. If you simply *must* have a burger and fries, get the smallest size possible.

Many restaurants are now catering to customers' demand for healthier choices, and most have nutrient information available if you request it. In general, smart low-fat choices include:

- Grilled chicken sandwich

- Grilled chicken or turkey salad

- Bean burrito

- Turkey, ham, or veggie sub

- Baked potato with broccoli and cheese

If you haven't already, make sure you purchase individual-sized servings of tuna, yogurt, yogurt drinks, low-fat cheese, small boxes of whole-grain cereal, and instant soups. Invest a few minutes each week to prepare foods you can grab and eat on the go. When you make dinner, make a little extra for the next day. Hard-boil a few eggs. Wash and slice veggies like peppers, celery, and carrots, and store in a container in the fridge. Keep a supply of healthy foods at work. Stash some nuts and dried fruit in your car. And if you are at a food court or need to hit the drive-through, know your healthiest options.

recipes

breakfast smoothies

A smoothie is a great breakfast on the go. You can make it the night before and store in the fridge in a to-go cup with a lid so you can dash out the door if you need to. Just shake well before drinking it.

banana–peanut butter smoothie   SERVES 1

1 cup nonfat vanilla yogurt

1 medium banana

1 tablespoon smooth, natural-style peanut butter

1 cup ice

Put all of the ingredients into a blender and blend until smooth.

Calories 363; Fat 8.7 g (Sat 1.9 g, Mono 3.9 g, Poly 2.3 g); Protein 14.2 g; Carb 60.7 g; Fiber 3.8 g; Chol 0 mg; Sodium 211 mg

strawberry smoothie   SERVES 1

1 cup frozen strawberries (about 6 berries)

1/2 cup nonfat vanilla yogurt

1/2 cup nonfat milk

1/4 cup cold water

Put all of the ingredients into a blender and blend until smooth.

Calories 166; Fat .7 g (Sat .2 g, Mono .1 g, Poly .3 g); Protein 9.5 g; Carb 31.0 g; Fiber 3.3 g; Chol 2.4 mg; Sodium 133 mg

apple crunch oatmeal SERVES 1

There are so many delicious ways to dress up oatmeal. This is one of my favorites.

1 cup nonfat milk

1/2 cup old-fashioned rolled oats

1/2 cup diced and peeled apple

2 teaspoons dark brown sugar

2 tablespoons low-fat granola

Put the milk, oats, and apple into a saucepan over a medium-high flame and, stirring frequently, bring to a boil. Reduce the heat to low and, stirring occasionally, cook for about 5 minutes or until the oatmeal reaches the consistency you like,

Transfer the oatmeal mixture to a cereal bowl. Stir in the brown sugar and top with the granola.

Calories 354; Fat 4.4 g (Sat .8 g, Mono 1 g, Poly 1.4 g); Protein 15 g; Carb 65.3 g; Fiber 6.3 g; Chol 5 mg; Sodium 161 mg

oatmeal 5 ways

Prepare your oatmeal with milk or soy milk instead of water to add protein, minerals, and vitamins. Regular oats are well worth the 5 minutes of cooking time, but if you need to, you can use plain, instant oatmeal instead.

PUMPKIN SPICE Stir in a dollop of canned pumpkin puree, plus a sprinkle of ginger, nutmeg, cinnamon, and brown sugar.

STRAWBERRY SWIRL Add sliced fresh berries, or thawed frozen strawberries with their juice, to your cooked oatmeal. Then swirl in a little strawberry jam for sweetness.

FRUIT AND NUT Add chopped dried apricots, dried plums, and raisins to your oatmeal as it is cooking so the fruit plumps up a little. Then add some toasted, chopped walnuts and almonds and a touch of honey.

BANANA WALNUT Top your cooked oatmeal with sliced bananas, chopped toasted walnuts, and a bit of honey.

OATMEAL COOKIE Add all the flavors that make oatmeal cookies so good: a drop of vanilla extract, some raisins, cinnamon, and a little brown sugar.

whole-grain blueberry pancakes SERVES 4

These hearty pancakes are a big treat on the weekends when you have a little more time to prepare breakfast. You can also make the batter the night before and store it in the refrigerator, so they will be quick to whip up the next morning.

$3/4$ cup whole wheat flour

$1/2$ cup all-purpose flour

$1/4$ cup cornmeal

2 tablespoons wheat germ

2 teaspoons sugar

2 teaspoons baking powder

$1/2$ teaspoon baking soda

$1/4$ teaspoon salt

2 large eggs

$3/4$ cup skim milk

1 cup low-fat buttermilk

$1/4$ teaspoon vanilla extract

1 cup blueberries, fresh or frozen

In a medium bowl mix together the dry ingredients (flour through salt). In another bowl beat together the eggs and skim milk, then stir in the buttermilk and vanilla extract.

Preheat a large nonstick griddle or skillet over a medium-low flame. Stir the wet ingredients into the dry ingredients, mixing only enough to combine them. Stir in the blueberries. (If you are using frozen berries, you don't need to defrost them.)

Ladle the batter onto the griddle or skillet, making any size pancake you like. Flip the pancake when it is golden brown on the bottom and the top is bubbling. Then cook the other side until golden brown. Serve immediately, or hold on an ovenproof plate in a 200°F. oven until the entire batch is ready.

Calories 283; Fat 4.5 g (Sat 1.4 g, Mono 1.3 g, Poly 1.0 g); Protein 13.1 g; Carb 49.2 g; Fiber 5.1 g; Chol 110 mg; Sodium 626 mg

ACTION

This week you'll establish a regular eating pattern, eating 3 meals and 1 or 2 snacks a day.

stretching

During the last two weeks, you've been walking three times a week. Now we're going to add one simple component to your fitness plan—stretching. It's a basic element of fitness, but one that most of us ignore.

why stretch?

Okay, be honest—when was the last time you felt flexible instead of stiff? At the end of the day, does your back ache or your neck feel stiff and sore? Do you notice little twinges when doing something as minor as bending over to tie your shoes? Unless you do yoga or stretch regularly, you've probably noticed that you're not as flexible as you used to be. While most of us neglect stretching, doing it regularly can help prevent injury, promote flexibility, maintain your range of motion, and serve as a great relaxation tool.

As you grow older, you tend to lose some flexibility, which makes you more likely to suffer an injury. For example, 80 percent of people suffer from back pain at some point in their lives. A stretching program can prevent common injuries and improve your overall flexibility—in one study, people who stretched for 30 seconds per muscle group each day increased their range of motion significantly in just a few weeks' time.

Taking just a few minutes to stretch several times a week can pay off in the way you feel throughout the day. Perform these simple stretches after warming up or after you've exercised—it's easier and more effective to stretch with nice loose muscles. Stretching when your muscles are cold and stiff, however, may make you more likely to suffer an injury. One of the simplest ways to incorporate stretching into your routine is to make it part of your cool-down routine.

six simple stretches

You don't have to perform a back bend or stand on your head to reap the benefits of stretching. In fact, some of the simplest stretches are also the most effective.

Remember to stretch after warming up or exercising when your muscles are looser and more flexible. You want to hold each stretch for three to five breaths. (I like to use breaths rather than counting because it helps you relax into the stretch.) Don't strain or stretch to the point of discomfort, and don't bounce while you're performing these moves. You want to stretch to the "edge"—you should feel a pull in the muscles you're targeting, but it shouldn't be painful.

Finally, don't get discouraged if you can't stretch very far when you begin performing these moves. Some people are more flexible than others, and you may progress slowly at first. Simply stretch as far as you can without pain—over time, you will notice an increase in your flexibility.

Triceps stretch

Stand with your arms over your head. Grasp your left elbow in your right hand and pull it toward your head, with the fingers of your left hand pointing down toward your spine. Feel a comfortable stretch in the back of your shoulder and upper back. Repeat with the arms switched.

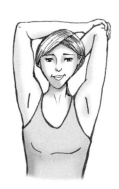

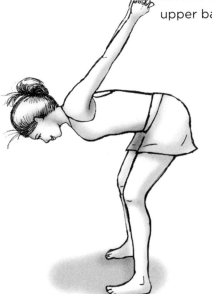

Chest/shoulders/hamstrings stretch

Stand and place your hands behind your back, with palms facing each other. With your feet shoulder-width apart, bend your knees slightly and lean forward so that your back is parallel to the floor, gently pulling your arms up toward the ceiling as you do so. When you feel a comfortable stretch in your shoulders and chest, straighten your legs as much as you comfortably can and extend the stretch to your hamstrings, the muscles along the backs of your legs.

Hamstring stretch

Sit on the ground with your legs in front of you. Bend forward and reach toward your toes—grasp them if you can, or hold your shins. (You can also wrap a towel around your feet and hold onto that while you stretch.) Without bending your knees, stretch forward as far as you can—you should feel it in your hamstrings and lower back.

Butterfly stretch (inner thighs)

Sit up tall and bring the soles of your feet together, letting your knees drop to the sides. Gently pull your heels toward your body and then press your knees toward the floor until you feel a comfortable stretch along your inner thighs. Grasping your feet with your hands, gently pull yourself forward by bending at the hips. If you want, you can press your elbows down on your legs to increase the stretch.

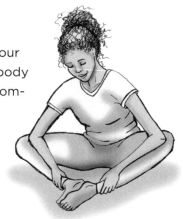

Quadriceps stretch

Stand with your hand on a wall or other stationary object for balance. Bend your right leg and hold your right foot behind your body with your right hand; gently pull toward your buttocks. Repeat on the other side with the left leg and hand.

Calf stretch

Stand facing a wall 2 to 3 feet away. Step your left foot about 18 inches behind you. Keeping your left leg straight, bend your right leg. Lean forward and press against the wall, keeping both heels on the floor—you'll feel the stretch in your left calf. Then repeat on the other side, stepping back with your right foot and stretching the calf muscle of your right leg.

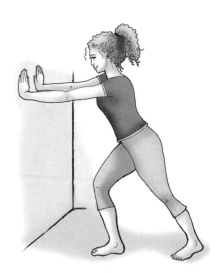

ACTION

Your action plan this week is simple. Continue walking 3 times a week at a low- to mid-intensity level. After your walk, perform the six simple stretching exercises.

managing your time

The number one excuse for not exercising? Lack of time. Today it seems like no one has enough time to do the things they really want to. Most of us carry around a mile-long to-do list every day and then spend weekends checking tasks off the list, only to have new ones spring up in their place.

You have only twenty-four hours in a day. If you always feel frazzled and it seems like you're spending all your time doing the things you *have* to do—and no time doing the things you *want* to do—it's time to learn how to manage your time better.

Does the idea of time management bring to mind complicated charts and having to track and account for every possible minute? Relax. You *can* prioritize and manage your time more efficiently in four simple steps.

step 1: take a look at your life

Figure out how you're spending your time. Consider how long you spend doing different activities in a typical day. You needn't account for every single second, but estimate how much time you spend on the activities below. You may find it helpful to track two weekdays and one weekend day for a more accurate picture of how you spend your time. You can record the time here:

ACTIVITY	DAY 1	DAY 2	DAY 3	AVERAGE
Getting showered/dressed/ready in the morning				
Eating breakfast/reading the paper				
Getting your kids ready in the morning (including making breakfast, taking care of lunch money, reminding about homework, driving kids to school, etc.)				
Commuting to work/working				
Preparing/eating lunch				
Preparing/eating dinner (and don't forget doing the dishes!)				

[CHART CONTINUES]

ACTIVITY	DAY 1	DAY 2	DAY 3	AVERAGE
Business-related activities				
Running errands				
Doing household chores (laundry, cleaning, paying bills, grocery shopping, yard work)				
Child-care tasks (helping kids with homework, playing games, separating dueling siblings, driving to soccer games)				
Watching television				
Reading (newspapers/magazines/books)				
Surfing the Internet/reading and sending e-mail				
Exercising/sports				
Spending time with your spouse/partner (talking, dinner out, sex, and "couple time")				
Charity/volunteer activities				
Socializing and spending time with friends/ family				
Sleeping				
Health/beauty (salon/doctor/dental appointments and the like)				
Hobbies/downtime				

Other activities: _____

step 2: consider your priorities

Now, make a list of your priorities, in order. (For most people, that's the tricky part.) Include children, spouse, other family members, friends, your job, your church, community or volunteer activities, exercise, having a clean house, watching a favorite television show, hobbies, sex, and the like. Put them in order as best you can:

MY PRIORITIES:

#1 _____

#2 _____

#3 _____

#4 _____

#5 _____

#6 _____

#7 _____

#8 _____

#9 _____

#10 _____

How'd you do? If you struggled with this exercise, you're not alone—most of us have a hard time deciding what's most important. Of course, your kids are your number one priority. But your spouse is important, too! And your parents and siblings. And your friends. And your career. And being financially secure. And having a nice-looking home. With all those competing demands on your time, it's no wonder a lot of us feel overwhelmed.

Obviously, some things will be priorities out of necessity. Your job may not be the most significant aspect of your life, but it's the way you put food on the table and provide for yourself and your family. That makes it important. Consider all the factors as you order (and possibly reorder) what your priorities really are.

step 3: **compare the results**

Okay, you've done the hardest part. Now take a closer look at the total amounts of time you're spending. How do they correlate to your priorities? If you work, you probably spend more time with your coworkers than your children. That may be unavoidable. But if you spend twelve hours a week watching television and one hour exercising—yet you say your "health" is one of your priorities—then it's time to reevaluate how you *spend* your time. (And by the way, how much time do you spend watching the tube? The average adult watches at least two hours a day, every day. Couldn't that time be better spent doing something else?)

step 4: **start making changes**

With your priority list in hand, look at the way you're spending your time, and consider ways that you can change your schedule. Can you group errands into one 2-hour block instead of doing them every day? Could you brown-bag your lunch and use the time to catch up on work instead of eating out every afternoon? If you spend hours driving your kids to and fro, could you consider a carpool? Do you really *have* to vacuum your house three times a week? (The answer—a resounding no!) Can you limit the television you watch to a few favorite shows instead of zoning out in front of it every night?

Check where you're overextended with your volunteer obligations as well. It's wonderful to contribute to causes you believe in, but many people overcommit themselves—at their own (and often their family's) expense. Come up with ways you can combine some of your priorities, like making a standing date with a friend to exercise together so you can get fit while you get caught up on your lives.

Start incorporating those changes into your daily life. It may mean asking your kids or your spouse for help. Are your kids old enough to start helping with household chores? Can your partner take over some of the errands on Saturday morning? Maybe it's better to turn down the chance at overtime to focus on the other aspects of your life right now. Remember, there will always be urgent tasks—paying bills, running errands, taking the car in to get the oil changed—that must be done. Don't be distracted by those and let your health, relationships, or well-being be the last thing you worry about. We all get the same 24 hours in each day. How you spend it, however, is up to you.

learning to say "no"

There's one magic word that can change your life, give you back your time, and help you lead a happier life. That word is *no.*

But I bet you have trouble saying "no," don't you? I know how you feel. You don't want to turn down that committee job for your son's school. Your daughter will be crushed if you're not the parent helper again this year. Your company always relies on you to organize the holiday party. Guess what. Sometimes you have to say "no"—to protect yourself, your time, and your energy.

But how? "No" seems like such a mean word. It's selfish, and you're not selfish, right? I've made your job easy for you—here are six ways to say "no" and not feel bad about it:

1. USE "NO, THANKS." Feel bad about saying "no"? Thank the person for the opportunity before you turn him or her down. "I really appreciate you thinking of me, but no, thank you." See? You can be polite and turn people down. (This works with phone solicitors as well!)

2. ASK FOR STALLING TIME. Too often we agree to do something on the spur of the moment. When asked for something, tell the person you need to think about it and you'll let her know. Then you can decide whether you want to take on the responsibility.

3. COUNTER WITH AN ALTERNATIVE. If you're not interested in the job or task but are willing to do something else, say so. "I'm sorry, I can't take on the chair responsibility, but I'm willing to help with the event the day of." (This is mostly a "no" but allows you to participate in something you want to without giving up your life for it.)

4. GIVE A REASON(S). Sometimes you have to say "no," and you've got a good reason—or ten of them—for doing so. If you're comfortable sharing them, let the person know—or say that you've been overextending your-self lately and need to cut back.

5. OR DON'T. "I'm sorry, but I can't." That's it. That's all you have to say. Yes, you'll feel guilty for a few minutes . . . but think how relieved you'll be afterward.

6. SUGGEST SOMEONE ELSE. You can't do it, but you know someone who might be interested? Pass along the person's name—it may be just right for him or her.

ACTION

Your action plan this week: start taking control of your time. Start saying "no" to things that don't fit your priorities.

WEEK 3
action summary

EATING WELL
- Shop to replenish your healthy pantry.
- Stay between 3 and 6 on the Hunger Continuum.
- Eat three meals and one or two snacks each day.
- Maintain your food journal.

GETTING FIT
- Walk for 20 minutes at low- to mid-intensity, three times.
- Add stretching to your walking routine.
- Note your walks in your journal.

FEELING GOOD
- Do the 5-minute breather daily.
- Practice a moment of mindfulness daily.
- Say "no" to tasks you don't want to and don't have to do.

WEIGHT_____

WEEK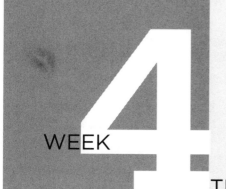

THIS WEEK'S CHANGES:

1. **Drink enough water and cut back on sugary drinks.**

2. **Add strengthening moves to your walking routine.**

3. **Create a bedtime ritual for better sleep.**

EATING WELL

you are what you drink

When you think "nutrition," the first words that come to mind are most likely vita-mins, minerals, carbohydrates, fat, and protein—all important nutrients. But the most vital nutrient is one that is often overlooked: water. For staying healthy and feeling your best, water works wonders. Even slight dehydration can cause fatigue, weakness, dizziness, and headaches. That's why getting enough fluid is a cornerstone of feeling well. But beyond basic hydration, studies show that water can help prevent condi-tions like kidney stones and urinary-tract and colon cancers. This week we are going to make sure you are drinking what you need to keep you at the top of your game.

how much is enough?

You have probably heard more than one nutritionist say you should drink eight 8-ounce glasses of water a day. While this is catchy advice, it is not completely accu-rate. Fluid needs are very individual. The amount you personally need depends upon your metabolism, your activity level, and the climate you are in. Plus, there are many beverages besides water that count toward hydration.

According to The National Academy of Sciences Food and Nutrition Board, most men need to drink about 101 ounces of fluid (13 cups) a day, and most women should aim to drink about 74 ounces (9 cups) a day. However, as your workouts get more intense in the weeks to come, and if you live in a hot climate, you may need to drink even more, depending on how much you sweat.

A good way to determine if you are drinking enough is to check your urine. Dark, scant urine generally indicates dehydration, while clear and frequent urine means you are on track. All those trips to the bathroom may be an inconvenience, but it is worth it.

options, options

You may be wondering how you will ever manage to guzzle that much water. Don't worry—you don't have to. Juices, milk, smoothies, sports drinks, and soft drinks all fulfill your fluid needs. Even drinks containing caffeine, like tea and coffee, and those containing alcohol count toward hydration. It is true that caffeine and alcohol are diuretics, which means they force your body to eliminate water. But at the end of the day our bodies compensate for the water loss, so caffeinated and alcoholic beverages ultimately contribute to total water intake.

Water, though, is the best beverage. It is absorbed quickly, it is calorie-free, and many studies show that water has an edge over other drinks when it comes to disease prevention. That's why it is a good idea to get at least half of your daily fluid needs in the form of water. That rounds off to 5 cups of water a day for women and 7 cups of water a day for men, as a minimum.

cut out the sugar

You can get the rest of your fluids from a number of different sources, as I mentioned. But clearly, all are not nutritionally equal. The most nutritious liquids are 100 percent juices, low-fat milk, soups, and smoothies. One hundred percent juices are packed with nutrients like vitamin C, folic acid, and potassium. Low-fat milk provides calcium and essential B vitamins. And soups and smoothies are also loaded with vitamins and minerals. All of these foods have calories, of course, so keep portions in mind.

Sodas, soft drinks, sports drinks, and juice drinks are excellent hydrators, but they are loaded with calories and lack the nutrients of 100 percent juices and milk. They are basically sugar-water. They make it all too easy to suck up hundreds of empty calories through a straw.

Take Charles, for example, a thirty-one-year-old investment banker from New York City, who came into my office completely perplexed. He was really pushing himself at the gym, he joined a basketball league, and he was eating very well—lots of vegetables, smaller portions, and no junk food. But despite all his efforts to trim down, he was gaining weight. He was very frustrated and about to give up. But I eventually discovered Charles's problem: he was drinking almost a gallon of cranberry juice cocktail every day! He figured he needed the fluid to rehydrate from his morning basketball game and thought he was making a healthy choice. He didn't realize that his "healthy" drink packed a whopping 1,300 calories! Charles didn't like plain water, so I suggested he try spiking his water with just a splash of the cranberry juice cocktail. Two weeks after making the switch, Charles came back, smiling, reporting a three-pound weight loss.

I have seen many cases like Charles's. Most people don't realize how quickly they can drink their calories, and when they cut back on sugary drinks, they almost instantly lose weight. That makes sense when you stop to think that a 12-ounce can of soda has 150 calories and the equivalent of about 10 teaspoons of sugar. You can lose half a pound a week simply by cutting out two sodas a day! Talk about the benefits of small changes!

Diet drinks are an option if you want your soft drinks without the calories, but I recommend using artificial sweeteners sparingly, so try to keep diet drinks to two a day. For flavorful, low-cal options, try adding a splash of juice and/or a squeeze of lemon to ice water or club soda. Herbal teas, served hot or iced, are also a good hydrating choice and many have a natural sweetness.

sports drinks

Sports drinks are also loaded with sugar, but they contain about half as much as soda and other soft drinks do. Their diluted sugar content plus the electrolytes they contain make them ideal hydrators. In fact, they are especially formulated to get water back into your body's cells rapidly, even more rapidly than water. But unless you are exercising intensely for over an hour, or in extreme heat, you don't need a sports drink. Save the calories. Water will quench you, and you can get all the electrolytes you need at your next meal.

tea

Herbal teas are delicious and caffeine-free and can have some wonderful healing effects. I use ginger tea to curb nausea, and mint and chamomile tea to aid in digestion. There are dozens of other herbal tea remedies, too many to get into here. But medicinal properties aside, herbal teas are tasty quenchers with zero calories.

tea time

The healing properties of tea make it a healthier alternative to coffee, and relaxing with a warm cup of tea somehow immediately calms you down. A special tea break is a wonderful way to escape the stresses of the day. If you have the time and inclination, consider making a little ritual of it. Use a nice teapot and teacup, break out the silverware and cloth napkins. Put on some soft music. Invite over a friend to chat, or just take some time for you. Sip slowly and enjoy. It is a healthy way to recharge, relax, and rehydrate, all at the same time.

Black teas and green teas have also been shown to have some remarkable health benefits. They contain powerful antioxidants called polyphenols, which have been shown to help protect your heart and guard against cancer. They also have an anti-bacterial effect. Keep in mind, though, that black and green teas do contain caffeine.

When drinking tea and coffee, also pay attention to fat and calories. Sweetened iced teas can have as much sugar and calories as soda. And a 16-ounce latte with whole milk tops off at 13 grams of fat and almost 250 calories—before you add any sugar to it!

calories and added sugar in beverages

DRINK	CALORIES	ADDED SUGAR (TEASPOONS)*
Water	0	0
Latte, skim (8 oz)	68	0
Milk, skim (8 oz)	86	0
Beer, light (12 oz)	100	0
Orange juice (8 oz)	112	0
Latte, regular (8 oz)	114	0
Wine (6 oz)	124	0
Sweetened iced tea (12 oz)	135–150	8–10
Soda (12 oz)	145–150	10
Beer, regular (12 oz)	147	0
Milk, whole (8 oz)	150	0

*I have included added sugar as opposed to the naturally occurring sugars inherent in the food.

alcohol

Most people I know jumped for joy when they heard the reports that alcohol has a protective effect on the heart. "Finally something seemingly sinful is good for me!" they cheered. In fact, a moderate amount of alcohol can be good for your heart health. Research shows that drinking any type of alcohol in moderation can lower

is too much joe making you jittery?

Are you one of those people who can't function without her first cup of coffee? Are you hooked on a mid-morning latte, or do you rely on diet sodas to keep you going through a long afternoon? While caffeine is the most widely used drug in the world, it can have some negative health consequences you should be aware of.

Caffeine boosts alertness and research has found that it can help ease headaches (that's the reason it's found in some pain relievers). It's also been shown to boost physical performance when taken before exercise. That's the good news.

The bad news is that as a stimulant, it may raise your blood pressure, and too much can make you jittery. Some studies suggest that it may contribute to bone loss, impair women's fertility, or be linked with headaches or chronic back pain. It also has a natural laxative effect and can cause heartburn and worsen ulcer pain.

What does this mean for you? As with most things, moderation is the safest bet. People's tolerance levels vary—you may be able to drink three cups of coffee with no ill effects while your friend is wired after a can of cola. But in general, it's a good idea to keep your caffeine consumption under 300 milligrams a day. (See page 85 for major caffeine sources.)

One note: if you decide to cut back on your intake, do it gradually to avoid possible headaches from going "cold turkey." If you're looking for caffeine-free beverages, drink herbal teas and decaf coffee and check the labels on your soft drinks. Many noncola beverages contain caffeine.

your risk of stroke, raise good cholesterol (HDL), and lower bad cholesterol (LDL). Red wine produces these positive effects, and more. It contains antioxidants that can further protect the heart.

That's all great news. But hold on, because once you drink past the point of moderation (which is defined as one drink a day for women and two for men), alcohol's benefits are quickly swallowed by its risks. Heavy drinking can really take a toll, leading to liver disease, stroke, cancer, and many other ailments. Alcohol also has plenty of calories. So if you don't drink, don't start. But if you do, enjoy. Just take it easy.

caffeine content of some popular beverages

8-ounce cup of coffee (brewed)	100–200 mg
8-ounce cup of instant coffee	60–85 mg
16-ounce coffee beverage	60–170 mg
8-ounce cup of black tea	25–50 mg
12-ounce can of soda	35–70 mg
12-ounce glass of iced tea	15–75 mg

recipes

spa water SERVES 4

They served this water at a spa I once visited, and I have been making it ever since. It really makes water special!

1 quart of cold water
1/2 cucumber, peeled and sliced

3 slices of lemon

Put ingredients in a pitcher and stir.

pink cocktail SERVES 1

Order this festive drink at a bar when you want to cut back on alcohol. Just ask for "club soda with a splash of cranberry and lime."

1 cup ice
1 cup club soda

1/4 cup cranberry juice cocktail
1 lime wedge

Pour club soda over ice. Add cranberry juice and a squeeze of lime, and stir.

Calories 37; Fat 0 g; Protein 0 g; Carb 9.6 g; Fiber .1 g; Chol 0 mg; Sodium 51 mg

Your action this week is to get enough total fluids every day, and make sure at least half of your fluid intake is water. For most people that means 9 to 13 8-ounce glasses of liquid total, including *at least* 5 to 7 glasses of water. Also, cut your intake of soda and sugary soft drinks to no more than one a day.

GETTING FIT
strength training

At this point, you've been walking 3 times a week and now are adding stretching after your walks. Believe it or not, you're already a quarter of the way through the program.

The next step is strength training. Even if you've never lifted a weight in your life, strength-building moves are an essential component of any fitness regimen. That doesn't mean you have to join a gym and start pumping iron—some of the most effective moves are ones you can do anytime, anyplace.

The objective of this week is to introduce the idea of strength training, and to show you how easy it is to incorporate into your fitness plan.

why strength train?

Cardiovascular exercises like walking, biking, and swimming are great for strengthening your heart, burning calories, and reducing stress. But they can do only so much to build and maintain muscle mass.

I know that you probably don't want huge, bulging muscles. But if you want a sleek, toned look—and a stronger, more injury-proof body—then strength training is for you. In fact, it should be an essential part of everyone's exercise routine: the American College of Sports Medicine recommends that adults perform at least one set of strengthening moves at least two or three times a week.

Does strength training bring to mind sweaty guys pumping iron in a gym? Relax. Simply put, strength training (also called resistance training or weight training) involves challenging a muscle (or group of muscles) beyond what it normally does. You do this using your body weight, free weights or dumbbells, exercise machines, exercise bands, or other equipment to provide resistance for the muscle to work against.

That effort creates microscopic tears in the muscle that are rebuilt by your body over the next couple of days. The result is denser, stronger, and sometimes—depending on how you train—bigger muscle. (If you're a woman, you need not worry about bulking up—professional bodybuilders train daily to achieve their eye-popping physiques.)

Not yet convinced? Well, strength training offers numerous benefits for both women and men:

It improves your appearance Cardiovascular exercise is great for reducing stress and burning calories, but it won't change the basic shape of your body. Nothing sculpts your body like resistance training—you must overload your muscles beyond what they normally do to tone them up. And firm muscles also help mask the appearance of cellulite by smoothing out those lumps and bumps of fat underneath the skin.

It boosts your metabolism Strength training helps make your body a more efficient fat-burning machine. Every pound of muscle you gain burns about 50 calories a day, even at rest, meaning when you have more muscle you can eat more and maintain your weight—or that you'll lose weight without changing your caloric intake. Because muscle weighs more than fat, you may not see the scale move as you build muscle and lose fat, but you'll notice that you look slimmer and leaner.

It keeps you young As you age, you begin to lose muscle and bone mass, but strength training can stave those off. Strength training helps maintain bone mass to combat osteoporosis. Strong bones also help you maintain good posture and make you less likely to suffer a fracture as you age.

It makes you tougher Not only do you look better, you're less injury-prone—the stronger your muscles are, the less likely you are to get hurt. (It is important to start off slowly with any strength-training program, as we are this week, to make sure you're not overdoing it at first.)

It reduces anxiety Studies show that strength training reduces anxiety and eases depression. At the end of a particularly crazy day, you may find that performing some strengthening moves helps you work off your tension. You're forced to concentrate on what you're doing instead of what's bothering you.

It improves your posture Those strong bones and muscles mean you'll walk taller. And not only will you stand straighter, you'll feel more confident as well—research shows that weight lifting improves self-esteem.

It makes life easier Strength training—duh—makes you stronger, so you're better able to perform functional tasks like carrying groceries or picking up your two-year-old. That makes you more efficient in your daily life, too.

Besides keeping you strong and healthy, strength training can radically improve your appearance. Many people focus on cardiovascular exercise, neglecting resistance training. Take thirty-seven-year-old Cindy, who'd been a treadmill junkie. She walked religiously but didn't notice a difference in her body until she added strength training to her program. She started a weight-training regimen several years ago, working out in the mornings before she went to work, and was pleasantly surprised by the results.

Within three months, Cindy could see a noticeable improvement in her overall physique. "I weigh the same, but I've lost inches," says the human resources professional who lives in Chicago. "I'm firmer and more toned. It's not like I've suddenly got huge muscles, either—it's just changed the shape of my body." Her arms and legs are slimmer, and now when she shops, she looks for sleeveless tops and shorts to show off her newly defined, sleek muscles.

seven super strengtheners

While some people work out with free weights (barbells and dumbbells), and others use weight machines at the gym, you don't need expensive equipment to get started. Some of the most effective moves—like pushups and crunches—simply use your body's weight as resistance instead of a machine.

These seven simple moves target your major muscle groups and will strengthen and tone you. Add them to your walking routine, after you walk and before you stretch. For a couple of these exercises, you'll need a dumbbell. But if you don't want to buy any equipment, take a look in your pantry: You can use a 16-ounce can, or put several cans in a plastic grocery bag.

Start with one set of 8 to 12 reps of each exercise, and concentrate on doing each move slowly—you'll get more results.

Modified pushups (targets chest and triceps, the muscles along the backs of your arms)

Start off facing down, knees slightly bent, hands at your shoulders, supporting your weight on your hands and knees. Keeping your body straight, lower yourself to a few inches off the ground and press back up. (If you're in good shape already, you can start off with your weight on your hands and toes, which makes it more difficult.) Do 8 to 12 reps.

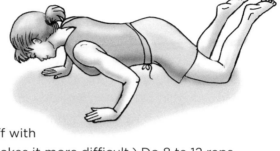

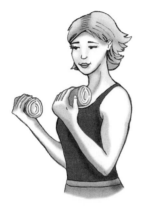

Biceps curls
(targets the muscles along the fronts of your arms)
Stand with feet shoulder-length apart, dumbbells (or cans) in both hands. With your arms at your sides, bend your elbows and bring your hands up toward your shoulders, keeping your elbows in and slightly in front against your body and your shoulders back, then slowly lower them back down. Do 8 to 12 reps.

Triceps kickbacks (targets the backs of your arms)
Stand and step forward with your left foot so that it's about 2 feet in front of you. Hold a dumbbell (or can or other weight) in your right hand with your arm bent, lean forward, and place your left hand on your left knee for support. Keeping your right upper arm tucked against your body, straighten your arm and then return to your original position. Do 8 to 12 reps and then switch sides and repeat with your right leg forward and working your left arm.

Back flys (targets the muscles of your back)
Bend forward at the hips, keeping your legs straight and knees relaxed, and hold a dumbbell or can in each hand. Keeping your body stable and your palms facing in, lift your elbows up and bring your arms up and away from your body, until your elbows are level with your shoulders, then return to your original position. Do 8 to 12 reps.

Bicycles (targets abdominal muscles)

Lie on your back, legs lifted off the floor, knees slightly bent, hands behind your head. Straighten and lower your legs toward the floor one at a time; as you do so, lift your head and shoulders off the ground and twist your right shoulder toward your left knee as the right leg lowers toward the floor and vice versa. Be careful not to bring in your elbows and pull your neck, just cradle it with your hands. Do 8 to 12 reps.

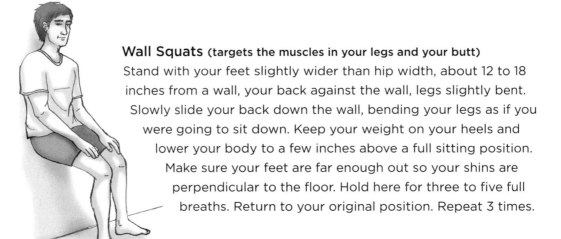

Wall Squats (targets the muscles in your legs and your butt)

Stand with your feet slightly wider than hip width, about 12 to 18 inches from a wall, your back against the wall, legs slightly bent. Slowly slide your back down the wall, bending your legs as if you were going to sit down. Keep your weight on your heels and lower your body to a few inches above a full sitting position. Make sure your feet are far enough out so your shins are perpendicular to the floor. Hold here for three to five full breaths. Return to your original position. Repeat 3 times.

Lunges (targets legs and butt)

Stand straight, next to a sturdy chair with your feet shoulder-width apart. Holding the chair for balance, step forward with your right foot, making a large enough step so that your shin stays perpendicular to the ground when you lower your body; push back up and return to your original position. Do 8 to 12 reps.

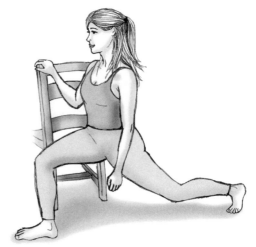

smart advice about dumbbells

While you can use a variety of equipment to do strength-building moves, you may want to buy some dumbbells to have at home. They're inexpensive and designed to be easy to grip.

Visit a sporting-goods store and experiment to determine which weight is right for you. (Start off with a light weight so you won't hurt yourself!) Choose a weight that you can do 10 to 12 repetitions with before you're tired; you may want to get two sets of dumbbells so you can use them for different moves. (Depending on the design, you may also be able to hold two in your hand once you're stronger.)

ACTION

Perform these strengthening moves 3 times this week in addition to doing your 20-minute walks and stretching. You may find it easiest to add the strength moves at the end of your walk, but feel free to do them at a different time of day (or even a different day) if you prefer. Just make sure you give yourself a day off in between the strengthening moves, to let your muscles recover.

FEELING GOOD
better sleep

I can't tell you how many times I've been asked by clients what kinds of foods they can eat for more energy or to improve the way they feel. When I interview them, I discover that they're sleeping only five or six hours a night (or less)—no wonder they feel tired! Sure, you can eat more healthfully, get more exercise, and reduce your stress levels, but if you're not sleeping enough, you're still not going to feel great. Simply sleeping more is often overlooked as a life-enhancing technique, yet sleep is essential for good health and a positive frame of mind.

Researchers still don't know exactly why people need to sleep every night. It may be that our brains replace necessary chemicals and get rid of toxins while sleeping, or that sleep is necessary to solve problems. When you don't get enough sleep, you begin to lose your ability to concentrate, think, and carry out even mundane tasks. You're also more likely to feel depressed or irritable.

The longer you go without sleep, the more pronounced these changes will become. There's something about the sleep process that helps restore the body and prepare it to tackle the next day. Research reveals that if you constantly short yourself on sleep, you'll weaken your immune system, which makes you more likely to get sick.

Yet most of us are chronically sleep deprived. According to a recent survey conducted by the National Sleep Foundation, more than half of Americans (63 percent) don't get the recommended eight hours of sleep per night. Nearly a third say they sleep fewer than seven hours a night. Not surprisingly, married people with children average less sleep during the week than those without children, and parents are also more likely to suffer from insomnia and more daytime sleepiness than nonparents.

how much do you need?

Researchers agree that the optimum amount of sleep for each person varies. Some people thrive on five or six hours of sleep while others feel better with eight or even nine hours. Babies, children, and teenagers need more sleep than adults. The amount of physical activity you perform can also affect the amount you need—you may need more rest after a strenuous day, for example.

You may already know how much sleep you need by judging from how you feel after sleeping different amounts. If you feel well rested after seven hours each night, that's probably your optimum amount. If you need eight and a half to feel human in the morning, shoot for that.

While most of us occasionally sacrifice sleep, remember that it will catch up with you. Sure, there will be times when you're unable to sleep or are up with a sick child or simply can't get your mind to stop racing. But by making it a priority, you'll set yourself up for a more restful slumber.

Getting enough sleep does more than just make you more clear-headed the next morning—it may make it easier to shed pounds as well. New research suggests that shorting yourself on sleep may make you hungrier and cause hormone alterations that affect your metabolism and make you more likely to gain weight. This makes sense—I see lots of people reaching for food when they're tired, hoping for an energy boost. What they *really* need is more quality time in bed.

sleeping better

It's not simply how many hours of sleep you get—it's the quality as well. If you constantly wake up during the night, you won't feel as rested in the morning. Less-than-stellar-quality sleep is a common complaint—seven in ten people say they experience frequent sleep problems. Yet there are a variety of ways to improve your sleep:

- Set a regular schedule. Try to go to bed and get up at the same time each day. This will help set your "body clock."
- Create a wind-down routine for yourself. If you've parented young children, you've probably done this with them to get ready for bed—first they put on their pajamas, then they brush their teeth, then it's time for a story. Create your own bedtime routine. That might mean taking a warm bath or curling up with a favorite book for a few minutes. Allow yourself time to wind down before you get in bed, and you're more likely to sleep better.
- Cut back on TV. The vast majority of us spend the last hour before bed watching TV several nights a week. If you're watching HGTV, that may be relaxing. Catching up on financial news or watching a violent drama may make you more prone to tossing and turning, though.
- Create a restful environment. Your bedroom should be dark, quiet, and a comfortable temperature—neither too hot nor too cold. If you have trouble sleeping, consider using your bed for only two things—sex and sleep. Using your bed to read, watch TV, or work may not be conducive to helping you sleep.
- Go easy on the alcohol—and sleeping pills. Alcohol makes you sleepy at first, but it reduces the quality of your sleep. Sleeping pills should only be used occasionally—they can be addictive and will produce insomnia once you stop taking them. While not a sleeping pill, melatonin has recently become popular as a sleep aid. Normally, your body produces this hormone when it's dark, and it appears to help regulate your body's internal clock. But researchers aren't sure what the long-term side effects of taking melatonin may be.

- Raise your body temperature—to drop it. There's some truth to a warm bath helping produce restful sleep—your body temperature drops after the bath, which makes you feel relaxed and sleepy.
- Exercise gently. If you crank out a workout a few hours before bed, it will probably affect your sleep quality because your metabolism will still be running high. Some light stretching or yoga poses are fine before bed, but perform your higher-intensity workouts earlier in the day.
- Eat lightly. A heavy meal late at night is likely to affect your sleep because your body's busy digesting it. A light snack is fine—milk or a carbohydrate snack will help relax you.

power napping

In some cultures, it's the norm to take a mid-afternoon siesta. That's when most people's energy levels dip. A short nap at this time can refresh and energize you for the rest of the day. A few tips on catching daytime ZZZs:

- Make yourself comfortable. That may mean stretching out on your couch or bed at home, or putting your head down on your desk at work.

- Make your area quiet. Earplugs can help drown out office chatter, or shut your door if you have one.

- Set an alarm. You won't enjoy your siesta if you're worried you're going to oversleep. Set your alarm clock or use a watch to wake you up.

- Limit your sleep time. A short nap—fifteen to twenty minutes—appears to be optimal. Sleep longer than that and you may feel groggy or find it harder to fall asleep later that night.

- Run it by your boss. You don't want to be caught napping on the job without clearing it with your supervisor first. Mention that you're going to cut your lunch break short and use the time to take a short nap later to help boost your productivity. How can she say "no" to that?

ACTION

This week, create a bedtime ritual for yourself. It need not be anything extravagant—just come up with a routine that will tell your body it's time to get ready for sleep. It might be washing your face and brushing your teeth before you climb into bed, or taking a few minutes to read before you slip under the covers. Set your alarm (if you use one) for the same time every morning, and try to get to bed at the same time as well—you'll sleep better in the long run.

WEEK 4
action summary

EATING WELL

- Shop to replenish your healthy pantry.
- Stay between 3 and 6 on the Hunger Continuum.
- Eat three meals and one or two snacks each day.
- Drink at least five glasses of water and no more than one soda or other sugary beverage each day.
- Maintain your food journal.

GETTING FIT

- Walk for 20 minutes at low- to mid-intensity 3 times.
- Stretch and do strength training 3 times.
- Note your exercise in your journal.

FEELING GOOD

- Do the 5-minute breather.
- Practice mindfulness.
- Say "no" to tasks you don't want to and don't have to do.
- Create a bedtime ritual.

WEIGHT _____

WEEK **5**

THIS WEEK'S CHANGES:

1. **Get enough healthy fat each day, and skip the bad fat.**

2. **Do something active just for fun!**

3. **Incorporate a mini-vacation or play break into your day.**

EATING WELL
the skinny on fat

Eat less fat. Stick to the right kinds of fat. Don't cut out too much fat. It seems like advice about fat—how much and what kind to eat—flip-flops with the seasons, leaving many people understandably confused and frustrated. This week, I'm going to clear up that confusion and show you how fat not only fits into a healthy and satisfying diet, but in fact is an essential component of it.

is fat bad?

In the 1980s, the major message coming from many nutrition experts was that fat is bad, and the less fat you eat, the better. The reasoning went that fat contributes to heart disease by increasing blood cholesterol. It also promotes weight gain since it packs more than twice the calories per gram (9 calories a gram) as carbohydrate or protein, which each have 4 calories a gram. Experts declared that fat is a big culprit in making America obese.

At the time, it seemed to make sense—eat fat, get fat. But our knowledge about fats has evolved in the past decades. We now know that simply reducing our fat intake won't necessarily make us thin. Americans, as a population, have managed to gain even more weight even after switching to low-fat cookies and fat-free ice cream. And we have discovered that while some kinds of fat are harmful, others are beneficial to your health and should be encouraged.

Just as no food is all "bad," fat shouldn't be considered bad either. In fact, it's an essential part of your diet. Fat makes food taste better, and can provide additional calories to those who need them. Your body needs fat to absorb fat-soluble vitamins, and it's also essential for healthy skin, hair, and cells. It also has some other important health benefits.

the good fats

However, not all fats are created equal. There are two main types of fats: saturated, which are solid at room temperature; and unsaturated, which are liquid at room temperature. As a general rule, the unsaturated fats are the healthy fats you want to be eating. Replacing saturated fats—those that come from animal products like meat, cheese, and eggs—with unsaturated fats can lower your cholesterol and protect your heart, as well as prevent other diseases.

Unsaturated fats are grouped into two categories—monounsaturated and polyunsaturated, each with its own positive qualities. Olive oil, olives, canola oil, peanut oil, avocados, cashews, and almonds are all foods rich in monounsaturated fat. This type of fat helps lowers bad cholesterol (LDL) while maintaining good cholesterol (HDL), and has been shown to protect against heart disease, stroke, and cancer.

Polyunsaturated fats come in two types—omega-3 and omega-6. Both are essential—you must obtain them from your diet to prevent a deficiency. Omega-3 and omega-6 fats are each critical to the health of all of our cells, especially those of the skin and immune system. But they play different roles in our bodies.

Omega-3 fat lowers bad cholesterol while keeping good cholesterol stable, and it helps reduce tissue inflammation, which is thought to be at the root of heart disease, stroke, and arthritis. Reams of evidence point to omega-3 as the healthiest fat, yet most of us do not get enough of it. The best sources of omega-3 fat are fish, especially cold-water fish like salmon, sardines, and tuna, as well as flax seeds and flaxseed oil. Walnuts also have omega-3 fat.

Omega-6 fat is a mixed bag. It is essential, and it lowers cholesterol when eaten in place of saturated fat. But it lowers both bad cholesterol *and* good cholesterol, and actually *increases* the inflammation that contributes to disease. Some big omega-6 sources include safflower oil, sunflower oil, corn oil, and mayonnaise made with these oils. Many foods, like walnuts, tofu, wheat germ, and soybean oil, are rich in both omega-3 and omega-6 fats.

Eating a mixture of the three types of unsaturated fats—mono, omega-3, and omega-6—is important. Most of us get more than enough omega-6 fat from salad dressings and cooking oils, especially when dining out. The key to consuming more healthful fats is getting more omega-3 and monounsaturated fats into your diet.

That means eating more fish, nuts, avocado, and tofu, including wheat germ and ground flax seed in your favorite foods (sprinkle them on yogurt or cereal, or put them in muffin and pancake batter), and using olive oil, canola oil, peanut oil, and flaxseed oil. (Keep in mind that flaxseed oil is very sensitive to light and heat, so you should not use it to cook with. Use it in salad dressings or drizzle it on cooked foods instead.)

the bad fats

Now you know the basics about the good fats. There are two kinds of fat that have proven health consequences and should be limited—saturated fat and trans fat. As I mentioned earlier, saturated fat is the kind found in foods like meat, full-fat milk and yogurt, cheese, cream, and butter. Saturated fat raises bad cholesterol and increases the risk of heart disease, stroke, and cancer.

Trans fat may be even worse for your heart than saturated fat, because it raises bad cholesterol *and* lowers good cholesterol. Trans fat is formed when oil is hydrogenated, or processed to become solid. Trans, or hydrogenated, fat is found in stick margarine, vegetable shortening, fried foods, and most commercially packaged baked goods, crackers, pastries, cookies, and many other products.

When hydrogenated fats like margarine and shortening were first invented, they were a boon to the baked-goods business. These new fats were solid like butter, so they made foods flaky and crisp, but they were much cheaper and more shelf-stable. They were also thought to be healthier than butter. That's why hydrogenated fat became the ingredient of choice and is rampant in the food supply. It was only recently confirmed that this fat is so unhealthy. Fortunately, manufacturers are now catching on to the idea that consumers want to avoid these harmful fats and are making efforts to reformulate their products to be trans fat–free. You can now find soft margarines that boast "trans-free" on their label, and many packaged baked goods are advertised as trans-free.

Starting in 2006, food labels will be required to list trans fat specifically. Until then, unless the food manufacturer has voluntarily noted trans fat on the nutrition facts panel, you have to do some careful label reading to determine if a food has it. Check the ingredient list for "hydrogenated or partially hydrogenated vegetable oil." The higher up on the list this ingredient is, and the more total fat that's in the product, the more trans fat the food has. Simply choosing low-fat baked goods can, by default, significantly reduce your trans fat intake.

You don't have to completely eliminate saturated fats like butter, fries, ice cream, and steak. Simply sticking to the "Usually/Sometimes/Rarely" lists (see page 233) will ensure that you get a good balance of the right kinds of fats. You'll see that on the list, I've designated the healthiest fats as "Usually" or "Sometimes" foods, and the not-so-healthy fats as "Rarely."

how much?

When it comes to health, it seems that the kind of fat we eat is more important than the amount. But healthy or not, all fats have the same number of calories, and those calories can add up quickly. So if you are watching your waistline, dipping your bread in a dish of olive oil may be healthy for your heart, but it won't necessarily help you stay trim. You don't need to walk around counting fat grams all day long, but having an idea of how much fat you should be eating each day, and becoming aware of the sources of fat in your diet, can help you make better food decisions that can ultimately help you lose weight.

I recommend eating a diet that contains a moderate amount of fat—about 30 percent of your total calories. To figure out how much fat you need, first determine your calorie range on page 237. Make a note of the calorie range you are in, because you will use it as a guide for the rest of the "Eating Well" changes in this book.

If you are in range I, you should aim for 40 to 50 grams of fat per day; range II, 50 to 60 grams; range III, 60 to 70 grams; range IV, 70 to 85 grams; and range V, 85 to 100 grams of fat each day. If you keep that number of fat grams in mind as your "ceiling," next time you check the label on a box of doughnuts, you might be inspired to skip it. Besides passing on the doughnuts, simple changes like switching to low-fat

bread spreads

To me, nothing beats the flavor of butter on my toast in the morning. But because butter is so full of artery-clogging fat, I use healthier, but still delicious, spreads most of the time and save the butter as a special treat. Some of my favorite toast toppers are peanut butter or almond butter and jam or honey, a smear of ripe avocado and a slice of tomato, or even a drizzle of olive oil and a little salt. I also love to make my Creamy Honey Walnut Spread. (See recipe on page 103).

If you want that buttery-ness without the bad fat, try trans-free tub or squeezable margarine. It isn't quite as healthy as the options I just mentioned, but it is a better choice than stick margarine or butter.

And if you need to reduce your cholesterol, try one of the cholesterol-lowering spreads like Take Control or Benecol. They contain compounds called plant stanol esters, and have been shown to reduce cholesterol by as much as 10 percent.

milk, yogurt, and cheeses, choosing extra-lean meats, and opting for low-fat baked goods can help you keep your fat intake in check. Get the fat you need from healthy food sources like nuts, fish, avocado, and tofu. These are all changes we will make in the weeks to come, so while you may incorporate them if you'd like, don't worry about them yet. This week's change focuses on *added* fat—the fat you put in or on food to make it taste better, as in dressings and spreads, and the fat that you cook with.

The box below gives you an idea of how much fat is in different foods.

how much fat is in that?

FOOD	AMOUNT	FAT (G)
Avocado	¼ avocado	8
Butter	2 teaspoons	8
Cheddar cheese	1 ounce	9
Chocolate chip cookie	1 small	4
Cream cheese	2 tablespoons	10
Egg	1 whole	5
Hamburger	4 ounces	23
Low-fat milk, 1%	1 cup	2
Margarine, soft	2 teaspoons	7
Nuts	¼ cup	18
Oil (all types)	2 teaspoons	9
Peanut butter	2 tablespoons	16
Salad dressing, regular	1 tablespoon	6
Salmon	4 ounces	13
Tofu	½ cup	5
Whole milk	1 cup	8

recipes

These versatile dressings are big on flavor but reduced in fat and calories. The fats they do contain are mainly the healthy monounsaturated variety.

citrus-ginger dressing SERVES 6

Try this dressing on a green salad garnished with sliced almonds and orange sections. Also use it in the simple flounder recipe on page 169.

1/4 cup orange juice

3 tablespoons lemon juice

1 tablespoon white wine vinegar

2 tablespoons canola oil

1 tablespoon honey

1 tablespoon peeled and freshly grated ginger

Salt and freshly ground black pepper to taste

In a small bowl, whisk together all of the ingredients until well blended.

Calories 59; Fat 4.6 g (Sat .3 g, Mono 2.7 g, Poly 1.3 g); Protein .1 g; Carb 4.8 g; Fiber .1 g; Chol 0 mg; Sodium .6 mg

balsamic vinaigrette SERVES 6

1/4 cup balsamic vinegar

1/4 cup olive oil

1/4 cup low-sodium chicken broth

1 tablespoon Dijon mustard

Salt and freshly ground black pepper to taste

In a small bowl, whisk together all of the ingredients until well blended.

Calories 90; Fat 9 g (Sat 1.3 g, Mono 6.6 g, Poly .8 g); Protein 2 g; Carb 1.4 g; Fiber 0 g; Chol .2 mg; Sodium 63 mg

mustard-dill sauce SERVES 4

This sauce is delicious for dipping raw vegetables. Also use it on poached salmon (recipe on page 169).

1/2 cup nonfat plain yogurt

2 teaspoons Dijon mustard

2 teaspoons lemon juice

1 tablespoon chopped fresh dill

In a small bowl, whisk together all of the ingredients until well blended.

Calories 20; Fat 0 g; Protein 1.8 g; Carb 2.6 g; Fiber 0 g; Chol 6 mg; Sodium 81 mg

creamy honey walnut spread SERVES 4

Use this satisfying spread instead of cream cheese or butter on toast or a bagel.

1 cup nonfat plain yogurt
1/3 cup shelled walnuts

2 teaspoons honey

Spoon the yogurt into a colander or strainer lined with paper towels or coffee filters. Put the strainer over a bowl and put into the refrigerator to drain for 2 hours.

Preheat the oven to 400°F. Spread the walnuts on a baking sheet and toast in the oven for about 5 minutes. Be careful not to let them burn. When they have cooled, chop them very finely.

Spoon the thickened yogurt into a small dish; discard the drained liquid. Stir in the walnuts and honey and serve.

Calories 110; Fat 6.6 g (Sat .7 g, Mono .9 g, Poly 4.7 g); Protein 5 g; Carb 8.9 g; Fiber .7 g; Chol 1.2 mg; Sodium 47.5 mg

roasted garlic SERVES 4 TO 6

Roasted garlic is one of the most versatile and delicious flavorings around. The roasting mellows the garlic and brings out a rich sweetness. I like to serve it as a bread-spread instead of butter or use it on sandwiches.

2 heads of garlic

1 tablespoon olive oil

Preheat the oven to 375°F. Remove the outermost papery skin from garlic and cut off the top quarter of the head so that the cloves are exposed. Put the garlic, cut side up, into a small roasting pan, drizzle with the olive oil, and cover the pan with foil. Bake in the oven for about 1 hour, until the garlic is soft and golden brown.

Serve the garlic head whole so guests can scoop the soft garlic out of each clove themselves with a knife and spread it on bread. Or squeeze the garlic out before serving it, puree it with a little more olive oil, and serve as a spread.

Calories 52; Fat 3.4 g (Sat .5 g, Mono 2.5 g, Poly .3 g); Protein .9 g; Carb 5 g; Fiber .3 g; Chol 0 mg; Sodium 2.5 mg

ACTION

Get two to four servings (depending on your calorie range) of healthy fats each day by cooking with them or using them on food. Reduce your intake of butter, stick margarine, fried foods, and packaged foods containing hydrogenated oil.

adding fun to fitness

This week, I want to talk about the importance of play in both your workout routine and your life in general.

fun + fitness = results

Think about the reasons you exercise. It may be to reduce stress, protect your health, or lose weight—or a combination of all three. But in search of achieving results, you may be forgetting that fitness can be *fun.*

If you're skeptical, bear with me. Physical activity can be enjoyable—you may have discovered by now that you like the feeling of walking or look forward to your thrice-weekly workouts as time for yourself. You may have found that even if you start your walk reluctantly, once you get going, you feel alive and invigorated. When you like what you're doing, you'll reap even more benefits—you're more likely to stick with your exercise program and you'll push yourself harder because you're more caught up in what you're doing. That means more results from your program.

Fun exercise (come on, it's not an oxymoron!) can also help change your mindset that working out has to be a difficult or boring chore. To get in touch with the joy of movement, watch young children at play. They're not worrying about burning calories or building strong bones or staying flexible. They're not putting in their required exercise time so they can check it off their mental list or log it in their journal. No, they're completely absorbed in what they're doing, whether they're zooming around as airplanes, jumping rope, or playing in a sandbox where they create cities of their own.

That rapt attention is what makes play so beneficial for children and adults both—during play, you can enter a state of flow where you're so focused on what you're doing that you forget everything else. In fact, flow is similar to a meditative state—the difference is that when you're performing an activity—playing the piano, practicing your tennis serve, or writing a novel—you're completely absorbed in the process.

adding fun to the mix

What does this mean for you? It means that the more you enjoy exercise, the less painful it feels, and the more likely you are to stick with it. After a few weeks, most people find that exercising becomes self-rewarding—they feel so much better afterward that they find it easier to keep up their routine. But if activity still feels like a chore, here are a few ways to inject some fun into your regimen:

From morning to night If you usually sleep as late as possible before crawling out of bed, get up early and walk first thing in the morning. If you usually exercise in the morning, opt for a lunch or early-evening workout instead. Simply changing the setting or the time of day you exercise can make a big difference in your attitude.

Tune into tunes Slipping on your Walkman can boost your workout as well. Choose some motivating music or pop in a comedy tape or CD—laughing will boost your endorphins as you exercise.

Change it up If you're bored with your walk, try a fun, different workout sometimes called *fartlek,* which is Swedish for "speed play." The idea is to add variety to your workout by mixing up what you're doing instead of going at the same pace. For example, you might walk as fast as you can between telephone poles, or jog for twenty steps every time you see someone walking a dog. Use this type of workout to add fun and spice to your walks—it makes the time go by much quicker!

Fuel your tank If you dread the idea of exercising, your body may be low on fuel. Have a high-energy snack an hour or so before your workout to fuel your tank. (See page 65 for high-energy snack ideas.)

Be social I've mentioned this before, but sharing an activity with a friend makes it more fun and makes the time fly by. Invite someone to come along with you, or sign up for a group activity where you'll meet new people.

Eye on the ball Playing sports like racquetball, volleyball, or tennis is a fun way to stay fit. When you concentrate on hitting the ball, you forget about what you're doing—you simply enjoy it. Feel free to substitute playing a sport for your walk, here and there, as you please.

Join your kids, or just act like one Grab your kids and spend an hour outside with them. Play tag, pickup basketball, or go for a bike ride together. It's a fun way to reconnect with your children and encourages them to be active, too. Or just act like a kid yourself. Grab the chalk and play a game of hopscotch, jump rope, or blast your favorite disco song and dance around your living room.

Try something new Just because you've been walking for four weeks doesn't mean you have to keep doing that. Try swimming, biking, or even Rollerblading instead—a new activity will help keep things fun.

ACTION

Add one fun element this week—like playing with your kids, going dancing, playing basketball, or roller- or ice-skating. That can take the place of one of your usual walks.

FEELING GOOD
the power of play

I've been talking about the physical aspects of play, but it has an emotional aspect as well. Play can be considered any activity that you find pleasurable or enjoyable. Given that broad definition, consider how often you play. Think you're too busy to have fun? Think again—play is crucial to our mental creativity, health, and happiness. Yet adults tend to forget about the importance of having fun.

Play can be anything that you enjoy—spending time pursuing a hobby, practicing a musical instrument, going bowling or shooting pool, or teasing your cat with a new mouse toy. The only requirement is that it's fun for *you*. Play is energizing and helps reduce stress; it may also help make us more creative.

8 easy stress-busters

Play is one great way to reduce stress, but there are plenty of others. Here are eight more proven ways to unwind:

STRETCH IT OUT. Sit in a chair and slowly hang forward, letting your arms dangle loose. This "rag doll stretch" helps release tension from the spine, neck, and shoulders and increases blood flow to the brain. It's particularly effective for helping you relax when you're exhausted.

TUNE IN. One of the simplest ways to de-stress is listening to music. Choose any music that you enjoy or that has special significance to you, and find a comfortable spot where you can relax, close your eyes, and really focus on it. You'll be transported from the stressors of the day.

SOAK IT AWAY. Run a tub full of water as hot as you can stand it, toss in a couple of chamomile tea bags, and "steep yourself" for twenty minutes. The effects of the hot water and chamomile will relax tense muscles.

GRIN AND BEAR IT. It may sound goofy, but it works—when you're feeling wrung out, smile and tell yourself that you feel fine and think positive thoughts. If that's too much of a stretch, think of someone you love and focus on that feeling. You can't experience fear, anger, or stress *and* love at the same time, so concentrating on positive, loving feelings can be relaxing.

FONDLE FLUFFY. Simply owning a pet may be one of the best ways to unwind—studies have shown that stroking or touching a pet reduces blood pressure. No time for a furry friend? Even watching fish can lower stress levels.

WRITE IT DOWN. Take a few minutes to record what's bothering you at the end of the day. Studies suggest that keeping a journal and writing about your feelings and ways to cope with difficulties can have a positive effect on your mood and help reduce stress.

GET RUBBED. Massage improves your circulation and relieves tension—and it feels fantastic, too! Schedule a massage at the end of an insanely busy week, or treat yourself after accomplishing something special.

WORK IT OUT. When your stress levels skyrocket, breaking a sweat is one of the best ways to fight back. A gentle walk may not have as powerful an effect as more intense exercise, though, so shoot for a 20-minute workout of about 70 to 85 percent of your target heart rate for more tension-reducing benefits.

laughter, the best medicine

Think how good you feel after a big belly laugh. It appears that laughing not only makes you feel great, it has emotional and physical health benefits as well. Researchers have found that laughter improves mood, reduces anxiety, eases stress, and is associated with creativity and emotional stability. It has physical benefits as well—laughter reduces pain, improves immunity, lowers blood pressure, and may contribute to a longer life, too.

Yet many of us don't take enough time to play—or we try to multitask to make the most of our "free" time. You agree to give yourself a few minutes to relax outside, but then take your laptop along to catch up on work. You're having lunch with a friend or playing some pickup basketball when your cell phone rings to interrupt you.

Carving time out of your schedule for play can seem self-indulgent, but its results make it worthwhile. That's why many businesses foster creative atmospheres where play is encouraged—research shows that employees who play feel happier and more relaxed and are more productive as well. Even a brief play break—a few minutes spent doing something fun or relaxing at work, for example—can serve as a mini-vacation that will add pleasure to your day while reducing stress.

ACTION

Your action this week is simple—incorporate a mini-vacation or play break into your day. You can use the 5-minute breather as your mini-vacation or experiment with other ways to add more fun to your regular daily routine.

action summary

EATING WELL
- Shop to replenish your healthy pantry.
- Eat regular meals and snacks, stopping when you are at a 5 or 6 on the hunger scale.
- Drink enough to stay well hydrated, including at least five glasses of water and a maximum of one sugary drink a day.
- Use healthy fats (two to four servings per day) for cooking, dressings, and spreads.
- Record in your journal everything you eat and drink.

GETTING FIT
- Walk for 20 minutes 3 times at low- to mid-intensity.
- Stretch and do strength training 3 times.
- Add a fun element to your workout at least once.
- Note your activity in your journal.

FEELING GOOD
- Do the 5-minute breather, or take a mini-vacation once a day.
- Practice mindfulness.
- Say "no" to tasks you don't want to and don't have to do.
- Keep up your bedtime ritual.

WEIGHT _____

WEEK

6

THIS WEEK'S CHANGES:

1. **Eat plenty of colorful fruits and vegetables.**

2. **Walk with more intensity.**

3. **Try deep relaxation or meditation.**

EATING WELL

the color of health:
fruits and vegetables

Think about all the outrageous claims marketers make about their pills, powders, and potions. This one is supposed to help you lose weight. That one will prevent aging and reduce your risk of disease. This one will give you more energy and provide your body with the vitamins and minerals it needs.

Yet none of these supposed claims could be more over the top than the *true* assertions you could make about fruits and vegetables. My ad for these "wonder-foods" would look something like this:

- Avoid killer diseases like heart disease, cancer, stroke, high blood pressure, and diabetes!
- Improve your memory and keep your brain sharp!
- Keep your skin healthy and reduce wrinkles!
- Prevent birth defects!
- Lose weight without hunger!
- Slow down your body's aging process!
- Delicious and satisfying!
- Available in unique color-coded packaging!

With that sales pitch, you'd think everyone would be eating their share of produce, wouldn't you? But the sad fact is that three out of four people do not come close to getting the recommended "five-a-day" servings of fruit and veggies. Why? Maybe it's because carrots and apples lack a billion-dollar advertising campaign. Maybe it's because your parents forced you to eat your peas when you were little and you vowed you'd never eat them again.

I encourage all my clients to eat plenty of fruits and vegetables. Yet during my years of private practice, I have heard all sorts of reasons why people don't, from "I just don't like vegetables" to "I buy fruit, but it winds up going bad in my fridge." This week, I'll enlighten you about the benefits of produce. Better yet, I'll give you some delightful and practical ways to get more fruits and vegetables into your life.

a nutritional powerhouse

Fruits and vegetables boast so many health benefits because they are loaded with nutrients—vitamin C, beta-carotene, folic acid, vitamin B6, potassium, magnesium, calcium, and fiber, just to name a few. They also contain a wealth of naturally occurring plant compounds called phytonutrients that act as antioxidants in your body—they neutralize substances (oxidants) that cause cell damage and are at the root of many health problems. All of this nutritional power makes fruits and veggies a mighty weapon against disease, obesity, and the effects of aging.

The only way to harness this power is to *eat* fruits and vegetables—despite what some pitchmen might claim, you can't bottle this stuff. Well, you can bottle *some* of it, but research shows that removing these nutrients from the fruit or vegetable that contains them reduces their effectiveness. Plus, since scientists are discovering new phytonutrients practically *weekly,* the only way to ensure you get all those wonderful phytochemicals, both discovered and undiscovered, is to eat your spinach . . . and strawberries and broccoli and oranges....

the color connection

How can you make sure you're getting the full spectrum of protective nutrients? It's simple—just eat a variety of different colors every day. Many phytonutrients impart color to food. For example, beta-carotene has a yellow or orange hue, and anthocyanins and lycopene are red. So don't worry about remembering any scientific names. All you need to do is fill your plate with a beautiful palette of color every day.

Red As I mentioned, the color red indicates the presence of lycopene and anthocyanins, which help you maintain a healthy heart, boost your memory, lower the risk of developing some types of cancer, and help keep your urinary tract healthy. Reds include strawberries, cherries, cranberries, red grapefruit, raspberries, watermelon, red apples, red peppers, pomegranates, beets, radishes, radicchio, red cabbage, rhubarb, and tomatoes.

Yellow/Orange Carotenoids give produce a yellow/orange hue. These foods help keep your immune system strong, maintain sharp vision, and lower the risk of heart disease and cancer. Go for apricots, cantaloupe, grapefruit, mango, papaya, peaches, oranges, pineapples, lemons, tangerines, yellow peppers, pumpkin, butternut squash, acorn squash, yellow summer squash, carrots, and other sunny colored produce.

Green Green fruits and vegetables contain lutein and indoles. Deep green vegetables are also loaded with key minerals like iron, magnesium, and calcium, plus an array of essential vitamins. Green foods help keep your vision sharp, prevent cancer, and maintain strong bones and teeth. Eat plenty of green apples, honeydew melon, green grapes, kiwi, limes, pears, avocado, asparagus, arugula, artichokes, broccoli, broccoli rabe, kale, collard greens, green peppers, green beans, lettuce, cucumbers, spinach, zucchini, green cabbage, and so on.

Blue/Purple These foods have anthocyanins and phenolics, which may have antiaging benefits. Try blackberries, blueberries, plums, dried plums, grapes, raisins, eggplant, purple potatoes, and purple asparagus to put purple on your plate.

White Many white and brown foods have powerful antimicrobial properties and many contain a phytonutrient called allicin, which has been shown to prevent heart disease and cancer. To reap these benefits, include white foods like bananas, dates, cauliflower, garlic, onion, mushrooms, ginger, parsnips, potatoes, shallots, and turnips.

the weight-loss factor

If all the health benefits aren't enough, fruits and vegetables can also help you lose weight. I have seen it many times. Once a person commits to eating more produce, the pounds come off. There are several reasons for this.

First, there is what I call the displacement factor. Your waitress asks you if you want fries or a side salad with your sandwich. Newly focused on getting your greens, you go for the salad. But at the same time, you're sparing yourself a couple hundred fatty calories (or more!) by opting out of the fries. Similarly, if you grab a banana for a snack, you are less likely to grab a cookie—and those "saved" calories add up!

Second, fruits and vegetables make you feel full yet they have very few calories, thanks to their high water and fiber contents. In fact, research shows that when your dish includes more vegetables, you feel just as satisfied with fewer calories. Adding more vegetables to your meals can produce slow but steady weight loss—that lasts.

21 ways
to get fruits and vegetables into your life

1. No time to make salad? No problem. Buy bags of prewashed greens and have a salad at the ready anytime.

2. Next time you are scrambling up some eggs, add some diced tomatoes, peppers, and onions for a veggie boost.

3. When dining out, make a habit of starting with a green salad.

4. For a simple yet special fruit dessert, arrange sliced apples and pears on a plate and sprinkle with cinnamon.

5. For a cool summer treat, keep blueberries and grapes in the freezer and nibble them while they are still frozen.

6. On your day off, make an extra-large batch of vegetable soup. Freeze the leftovers in single-serving containers for an instant homemade veggie fix on a busy day.

7. Add fruit to your salad. Orange and grapefruit sections, apple and pear slices, grapes, raisins, and even strawberries add a juicy burst of flavor and color.

8. Go beyond lettuce and tomato and add extra veggies to your sandwich. Try slices of pepper, cucumber, avocado, or grated carrot on your sandwich. Pita bread is great for holding lots of veggies.

9. Stash some dried fruit—apricots, raisins, dried plums, dried apples, dates—in your desk drawer or glove compartment. Enjoy with a handful of nuts for an energizing snack.

10. Toss a handful of chopped broccoli or fresh or frozen spinach into your pasta sauce as you heat it.

11. Every Monday, bring five pieces of fresh fruit to work and keep them in a basket on your desk. Not only will you eat more fruit, you'll also enjoy how it looks!

12. Give your tuna salad a colorful, crunchy kick: add chopped celery, onion, peppers, and carrots.

13. When grilling, try marinated vegetable kebobs. Just skewer mushrooms, cherry tomatoes, peppers, and onions, marinate in olive oil and vinegar, and grill.

14. Fresh fruit is also delicious on the grill—especially sliced pineapple and peach halves. Just brush with a little oil and grill until warm. Serve with a bit of frozen yogurt and some mint.

15. At a cocktail party, try a Virgin Mary, plain tomato juice, or club soda with a splash of orange juice for a vitamin-packed, alcohol-free alternative.

16. Don't settle for plain pancakes. Toss some berries or sliced banana in the batter.

17. Keep a bag of baby carrots at home and in the fridge at the office for a handy crunchy-munchy.

18. For a satisfying snack, spread some peanut butter on apple halves or on a banana.

19. Top off a romantic dinner with a luscious, romantic fruit like strawberries or cherries. For maximum sex appeal, feed them to each other!

20. If you cut it, it will go. Take a half hour each week to cut up fresh fruit and veggies and store them in sealed containers. Whole melons and unpeeled fruit might rot in your refrigerator, but no one can resist a ready-to-eat fruit salad. And peppers, celery, and carrots are much more enticing when they are already washed and cut.

21. Visit your local farmers market. You'll be amazed at the array of colorful, delicious produce you'll find. Go out on a limb and try something you've never had before.

how much is enough?

The American Dietetic Association recommends a minimum of five servings of fruits and vegetables every day. Personally, I recommend two to four servings of fruit and three to six servings of vegetables a day. That may sound like a lot, but remember that the suggested serving sizes are small—most of us can easily eat several servings at a meal. Check your calorie range on page 237 to see how many servings you should aim for.

One small whole fruit, 1 cup berries or fresh fruit salad, $\frac{1}{2}$ cup canned fruit salad, $\frac{1}{4}$ cup dried fruit, and $\frac{3}{4}$ cup fruit juice each count as a serving of fruit. And one serving of vegetables is $\frac{1}{2}$ cup cooked vegetables, $\frac{1}{2}$ cup chopped raw vegetables, 1 cup salad greens, or $\frac{3}{4}$ cup vegetable juice. So a 6-ounce (diner-sized) glass of OJ at breakfast and an apple in the afternoon can cover your minimum fruit quota, and a handful of baby carrots at lunch and a cup of cooked broccoli can get you up to par on veggies for the day.

As far as upper limits go, it is nearly impossible to eat too many vegetables. So although I recommend three to six servings as the range to shoot for, enjoy as many vegetables as you care to. I have seen people go overboard on fruit, though, eating it at the expense of other healthful foods, or consuming so much that they add significant calories to their diet. With this in mind, try to keep fruit servings to no more than four a day. Pay special attention to fruit juice—while it's a fine way to consume fruit, it's easy to gulp down too much. A juice-bar "small" size is usually about 16 ounces—that's four servings of fruit right there. Also, when you drink juice, you miss out on valuable fiber. So choose the whole fruit whenever possible.

no ifs, ands, or buts

As I mentioned, three out of four people don't get the recommended servings of fruits and vegetables. If you are one of that majority, now is the time to make a change. You say you simply hate vegetables? Go back to the shopping list on pages 30–31 and circle any vegetable that you even remotely like—or that you haven't tried. Even the most ardent vegetable haters can find two or three vegetables they enjoy. Once you find them, make sure you always have them on hand.

Also, make an effort each week to try one new veggie, or a new way of cooking or preparing it. Some of your dislike may be from past prejudices, or assumptions from childhood. Our tastes can change—give yourself a chance to find out. For example, you may detest cooked spinach but enjoy a spinach salad. And veggies like carrots can be eaten raw, served with a low-fat dip or dressing, cooked with a little brown sugar, or used in soup.

Sneaking vegetables into foods you already like is another option. Stir a tablespoon of canned pumpkin into your oatmeal, add finely grated carrot to your pasta sauce, or add extra vegetables to your chicken noodle soup. Also try my macaroni and cheese recipe on page 137. It sneaks in a healthy serving of winter squash. If you find that fresh produce winds up spoiling before you get to it, no problem:

frozen and canned produce are other healthy choices, and an easy way to keep fruits and veggies at your fingertips. Stock up on frozen spinach, peas, corn, broccoli, squash, and fruit. Vegetable medleys make for a quick and easy stir-fry, and frozen fruit whips up in no time for a frothy smoothie. Canned tomatoes, pumpkin, corn, peas, pineapple, and mandarin oranges are staples in my cupboard. Whenever possible, opt for low-sodium varieties and fruit in its own juice, rather than in syrup, to keep salt and sugar consumption low.

recipes

summer vegetable sauté SERVES 4

This simple crowd pleaser makes the most of summer's produce. It tastes best when you get your ingredients from a local farmstand.

4 large ears of corn (or 2 cups frozen corn kernels, thawed)

1 tablespoon olive oil

1 large onion, diced (about 2 cups)

1 medium zucchini, cut in half lengthwise, then sliced (about 2 cups)

2 medium tomatoes, coarsely chopped (about 2 cups)

¼ cup chopped basil leaves

Salt and freshly ground black pepper to taste

If using fresh corn, husk it and remove the corn from the cob by holding the corn at an angle over a large bowl and cutting along the ear with a sharp knife.

Heat the oil in a large nonstick skillet over a medium-high flame. Add the onion and cook for 3 minutes. Add the zucchini and corn and cook for 3 minutes more, stirring occasionally. Add the tomatoes and basil and cook for 2 minutes more. Season with salt and pepper to taste.

Calories 189; Fat 5 g (Sat .7 g, Mono 2.9 g, Poly 1 g); Protein 5.5 g; Carb 36.5 g; Fiber 5.7 g; Chol 0 mg; Sodium 252 mg

sesame-orange spinach SERVES 4

2 bunches fresh spinach (about 1¹/₂
    pounds)
1 tablespoon canola oil
2 tablespoons low-sodium soy sauce
1 tablespoon lemon juice

2 oranges, peeled and separated into
    sections
¹/₂ teaspoon sesame oil
1 tablespoon toasted sesame seeds

Trim the stems from the spinach, wash it thoroughly, and pat it dry with paper towels or spin in a salad spinner. Chop it slightly.

In a large nonstick skillet, heat the oil over a medium flame. Add the spinach in 2 or 3 batches, cooking each batch until the leaves are wilted. When all the spinach has wilted, stir in the soy sauce and lemon juice and let simmer for about 3 minutes.

Chop the orange sections into bite-sized pieces. Add them to the spinach and cook for 1 more minute. Stir in the sesame oil and sprinkle with sesame seeds.

Calories 101; Fat 5.6 g (Sat .5 g, Mono 2.6 g, Poly 1.7 g); Protein 6.2 g; Carb 9.6 g; Fiber 16.7 g; Chol 0 mg; Sodium 502 mg

creamy cauliflower soup SERVES 6

1 large head cauliflower
1 tablespoon olive oil
1 medium onion, sliced (about 1 cup)
2 medium potatoes, diced (about 1¹/₂
    cups)

48-ounce can of low-sodium chicken broth
    or vegetable broth
Salt and freshly ground black pepper to
    taste
Nutmeg to taste

Cut the stem off the cauliflower and break it up into flowerets.

In a soup pot, heat the olive oil over a low-medium flame. Add the onion, reduce the heat to low, and cook until golden brown, about 10 minutes, stirring occasionally. Stir in the potato. Add the cauliflower and broth and bring to a boil over a medium heat. Reduce the heat to low and let simmer until the cauliflower is very tender, about 20 minutes. Add salt and pepper to taste.

Transfer to a blender or use a hand blender and puree until smooth. Sprinkle with nutmeg before serving.

Calories 102; Fat 2.9 g (Sat .4 g, Mono 1.8 g, Poly .4 g); Protein 6.5 g; Carb 14.2 g; Fiber 6 g; Chol 0 mg; Sodium 410 mg

balsamic swiss chard SERVES 4

Swiss chard is one of my favorite green leafy vegetables. But you can substitute spinach or kale in this recipe.

1 large bunch Swiss chard (about 1¹/₂ pounds)

1 tablespoon olive oil

1 garlic clove, minced

3 tablespoons low-sodium chicken broth

1 tablespoon balsamic vinegar

Salt and freshly ground black pepper to taste

Wash the Swiss chard thoroughly. Tear the leaves from the thick stalks, chop the stalks into small pieces, and put aside. Then cut the leaves crosswise into ¹/₂-inch-wide ribbons.

Heat the oil in a large pot over a medium-low flame. Add the chopped stalks and sauté for about 2 minutes, until they soften slightly. Stir in the garlic and sauté for 1 minute more. Add the leaves and stock. Cover and cook for about 4 minutes. Add the vinegar and salt and pepper to taste.

Calories 70; Fat 3.8 g (Sat .5 g, Mono 2.6 g, Poly .4 g); Protein 3.3 g; Carb 7.8 g; Fiber 2.7 g; Chol .2 mg; Sodium 370 mg

chopped salad SERVES 4

This dish shows how you can turn your usual salad ingredients into something really special simply by cutting them differently and adding fresh herbs.

1 head romaine lettuce, finely chopped

2 medium tomatoes, finely chopped (about 2 cups)

1 green, yellow, or red bell pepper, finely chopped (about 1 cup)

1 cucumber, peeled, seeded, and finely chopped (about 1¹/₂ cups)

¹/₃ cup finely chopped fresh basil leaves

¹/₂ cup chopped, pitted kalamata olives

2 tablespoons olive oil

2 tablespoons red wine vinegar

Salt and freshly ground black pepper to taste

Combine the lettuce, tomatoes, peppers, cucumber, basil, and olives in a large bowl. Drizzle on the olive oil and vinegar and toss. Season with salt and pepper to taste.

Calories 120; Fat 8.3 g (Sat 1 g, Mono 5 g, Poly .8 g); Protein 2.8 g; Carb 10.5 g; Fiber 3.5 g; Chol 0 mg; Sodium 275 mg

mango salsa SERVES 6

This is a colorful way to spice up simply grilled or broiled fish or chicken. Just spoon some on top of the fillet once it is cooked and serve. It is also delicious as a party food, scooped up with baked corn chips.

1 ripe mango, diced
1/2 avocado, diced
1/2 cup diced red onion
1/3 cup chopped cilantro

1 tablespoon freshly squeezed lime juice
1 tablespoon finely diced jalapeño pepper, or to taste
Salt to taste

Toss together all the ingredients in a medium mixing bowl. Serve at room temperature or chilled. Store covered in the refrigerator for up to 2 days.

Calories 55; Fat 2.6 g (Sat .4 g, Mono 1.6 g, Poly .3 g); Protein .7 g; Carb 8.5 g; Fiber 1.7 g; Chol 0 mg; Sodium 5 mg

peach crisp SERVES 8

Cooking spray
5 cups sliced, peeled peaches (thawed, if frozen)
1/4 cup orange juice
1/3 cup whole wheat flour

1/2 cup packed brown sugar
1 cup regular oats
1/2 cup chopped pecans
1/4 cup canola oil
1/2 teaspoon ground cinnamon

Preheat the oven to 375°F. and coat an 8-by-8-inch baking pan with cooking spray.

Toss the peaches and orange juice in a medium bowl, then spoon into the prepared baking pan.

In a medium bowl, combine the flour, sugar, oats, pecans, oil, and cinnamon. Stir with a fork until crumbly. Sprinkle the mixture over the peaches. Bake for 35 to 40 minutes, or until the topping is crisp and the peaches are tender.

Calories 245; Fat 12.5 g (Sat 1 g, Mono 7 g, Poly 3.7 g); Protein 3.7 g; Carb 33.2 g; Fiber 4 g; Chol 0 mg; Sodium 4 mg

poached pears in red wine sauce SERVES 4 TO 6

1½ cups red wine
½ cup brown sugar
1 tablespoon freshly squeezed lemon juice

1 cinnamon stick
4 ripe but firm Bartlett or Bosc pears
1 teaspoon vanilla extract

In a saucepan, combine the wine with 1 cup water and the sugar, lemon juice, and cinnamon. Bring to a gentle boil, stirring to dissolve the sugar. Lower the heat and let the sauce simmer for 10 minutes.

In the meantime, peel and core the pears and cut them into quarters. Add the pears to the hot liquid, cover, and cook gently for 20 to 25 minutes, until the pears are tender.

Transfer the pears to a dish using a slotted spoon.

Boil the liquid, uncovered, until it is reduced to about 1 cup. Stir in the vanilla. Spoon the sauce over the pears, cover, and refrigerate until ready to serve. Serve chilled.

Calories 233; Fat .7 g (Sat 0 g, Mono .1 g, Poly .2 g); Protein .8 g; Carb 44.6 g; Fiber 4 g; Chol 0 mg; Sodium 12 mg

ACTION

Eat *at least* two servings of fruit and three servings of vegetables every day.

GETTING FIT
speeding up

You're beginning Week 6, which means you're nearly halfway through the program! At this point, you're walking regularly and doing strengthening and stretching exercises 3 times a week. This week I'm going to focus on intensity and show you how to make walking or any other cardiovascular exercise more challenging—and increase the benefits you get from it.

what is that woman doing, anyway? other walking techniques

If you spend time outside, you've probably seen someone "race walking" or "power walking." Race walkers don't just walk—they walk *fast*. They swivel their hips and pump their arms as they walk to achieve maximum speed. (I know, it looks silly—but it's a killer workout!)

Power walking is a more generic term that can describe any kind of walking done at a more aggressive pace than an easy stroll. Power walkers take on additional obstacles like hills to make their walks tougher, or use weighed vests, hand weights, or even walking poles to increase the intensity of the workout. (By the way, please don't walk with ankle weights on—you're much more likely to suffer an injury. If you want to up the intensity, light hand or wrist weights or weighted vests are a safer option.)

Finally, there's running or jogging. Actually, walking at a fast pace burns as many calories per minute as slow jogging, so there's no reason to run unless you want to. If you're new to exercise, though, a walking routine is safer—there's less pounding and impact on your feet and legs. (I'll show you how to start jogging in Week 10.)

why walk faster?

Back in Week 2, I introduced you to the idea of exercise intensity. Remember that in this program we use three levels of intensity:

- **Level 1: Low-Intensity Walking** is relatively slow, yet purposeful walking. This type of exercise helps to build stamina and cardiovascular strength and serves as an excellent fitness walk for beginners. Low-intensity walkers average about 3 miles per hour and cover 1 mile in about 20 minutes.
- **Level 2: Mid-Intensity Walking** is a brisker-paced walk where the walker typically moves at about 4 miles per hour, covering a mile in about 15 minutes.
- **Level 3: High-Intensity Walking** is very fast walking that may include periods of jogging or running where walkers zip along at about 5 miles per hour, covering a mile in about 12 minutes. This form of walking is great for burning calories and toning muscles.

This week, you'll take your walking up a notch by increasing the intensity of what you do. Don't worry—you've already got five weeks of regular training under your belt, so you should be ready for this next level. In fact, you may feel that your walks have started to feel too easy or that you've increased your walking speed without even meaning to.

Do you remember from Week 2 that there are three basic ways to make exercise more challenging? You can increase the amount of time you exercise, increase the number of times each week you exercise, or increase your speed or effort level. All place additional challenges on your body, which helps you become fitter.

Why bother to do this? Because without increasing the intensity or the challenge placed on it, your body adjusts to the demands being placed on it and plateaus. Walking 3 times a week for 20 minutes will improve your fitness if you're sedentary, but who wants the bare minimum? Upping your intensity will increase the amount of rewards you receive from exercise as well. Make it a little bit harder and you make the payoff bigger, too.

You have three ways to make your walk more challenging. Pick one to add a little extra challenge to your walks this week—or try each:

■ Walk for 30 minutes (instead of 20).
■ Walk for 20 minutes at a faster pace (about 10 percent faster than you usually walk).
■ Walk for 20 minutes at your current pace, but do it up and down hills (or use an incline setting on the treadmill) to increase your effort.

ACTION

Your basic exercise routine stays the same—you'll continue walking 3 times this week and performing your strength and stretching exercises, but you'll up the intensity of your walks.

meditation

meditation: **the fast track to relaxation**

Over the past five weeks, you've been paying more attention to the way you breathe with the 5-minute breather exercise. You may have noticed that you're more aware of your inhalations and exhalations, and discovered that simply slowing down and focusing on your breath help you relax. This week we'll take that relaxing effect a step further and explore meditation.

Meditation is difficult to describe, but it's considered an alert, focused state of mind where you are aware of what is happening around you without losing yourself in thoughts or daydreams. Usually people meditate by sitting quietly and focusing on their breath, or a word or phrase, but meditation can also be performed walking or standing. It's a way of quieting that internal chatter that you probably hear all day. When you meditate, you lower your blood pressure and heart rate and you reduce stress—those physical benefits are what attract many people to meditation. It also reduces the amount of cortisol and other stress hormones your body produces, which may help prevent weight gain.

Meditation is basically a form of mental self-control. It occurs when your mind is so focused on what you're doing that you're not aware of anything else. There are a variety of ways to meditate, and I've included several below.

Breathing meditation This is one of the simplest ways to meditate, and is a natural progression from the 5-minute breather exercise. Choose a quiet place and sit comfortably. (Don't lie down—you may wind up falling asleep.) Breathe slowly, and count your breaths as you exhale: "inhale—one; inhale—two; inhale—three; inhale—four," and then start over at one. Focus only on your breath, and try not to lose count.

If you do lose count, or you find yourself thinking about other things, simply return your focus to your breathing. Don't worry about how many times you lose track or are distracted by other thoughts—simply sit and imagine those thoughts floating away. You may be surprised at how difficult you find this, especially at the beginning. Try setting a timer or stopwatch for 10 minutes, and work your way up to 20 minutes of meditation.

Word meditation Sit comfortably in a quiet place, and repeat a word or phrase over and over to keep your mind from wandering. You might use a word like *relax, calm, peace,* or *still.* If your mind strays, simply return to your word and concentrate on it.

Heartbeat meditation Sit comfortably, with your hand over your heart or fingers over your pulse. After you locate your heartbeat, sit and count each beat to 4, like you would with your breath. If you lose track, simply start over.

i didn't know it would be so hard!

As I mentioned above, meditation is surprisingly difficult for most people. You may find it impossible to quiet your mind, to stop thinking of all the (more important) things you could be doing while you're sitting there trying to meditate. Or you may feel frustrated that you can't do it. Try not to let emotions intrude while you're meditating—if you think of something else, simply bring your attention back to your breath, or the word you're repeating, or your heartbeat.

Remember, too, that you're not competing with anyone else as you meditate. You're not being graded on your performance—you're simply exploring a new way to quiet your mind and achieve greater serenity. Try it several times before you decide it's not for you—the more you do it, the easier it becomes to slip into a deeply relaxed, meditative state.

ACTION

Experiment with meditation by doing a meditation exercise for 10 to 15 minutes at least once this week.

action summary

EATING WELL
- Shop to replenish your healthy pantry.
- Eat regular meals and snacks, stopping when you are at a 5 or 6 on the hunger scale.
- Drink enough to stay well hydrated, including at least five glasses of water and a maximum of one sugary drink a day.
- Use healthy fats for cooking, dressings, and spreads.
- Eat two to four servings of fruit and three to six servings of vegetables each day.
- Record in your journal everything you eat and drink.

GETTING FIT
- Walk for 20 to 30 minutes 3 times at mid-intensity.
- Stretch and do strength training 3 times.
- Add a fun element to your fitness program.
- Note your activity in your journal.

FEELING GOOD
- Do the 5-minute breather or mini-vacation once a day.
- Practice mindfulness.
- Say "no" to tasks you don't want to and don't have to do.
- Keep up your bedtime ritual.
- Do a deep-relaxation or meditation exercise at least once.

WEIGHT _____

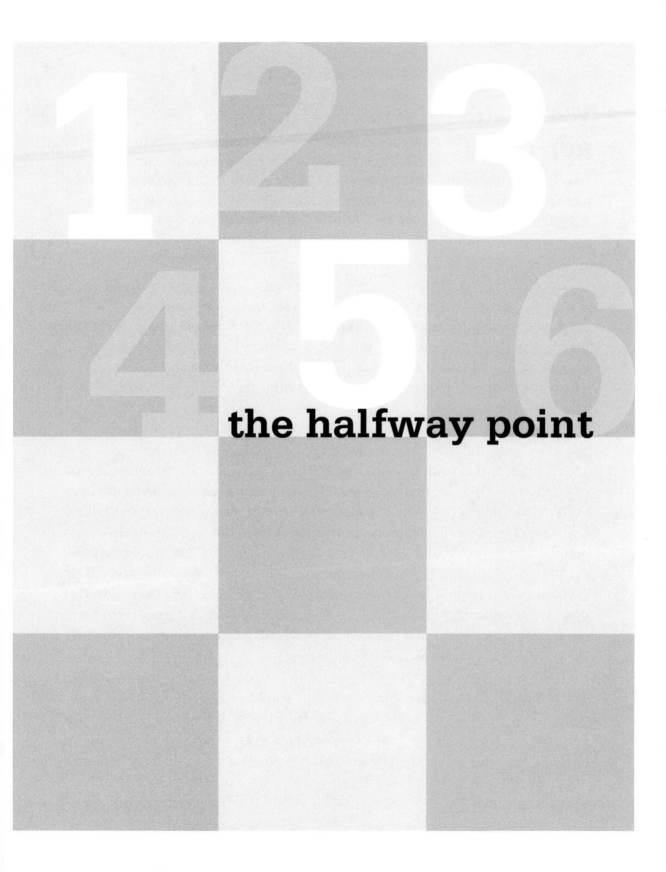

the halfway point

You're halfway there! Congratulations!

Look how far you've come. First, your diet has improved—at this point, you're keeping "Usually" foods on hand, eating intuitively, eating regularly throughout the day, and consuming the right amounts and kinds of fats, fluids, fruits, and vegetables. In the weeks to follow, you'll learn more ways to improve the way you eat and reach your nutritional goals, whether it's to lose weight, be healthier, or have more energy—or all of the above!

Fitness-wise, you've established a regular workout program of walking 3 times a week for 20 to 30 minutes at mid-intensity, and you're performing stretching and strengthening exercises as well. Best of all, you've learned how to make fitness fun. For the remainder of the program, you'll learn ways to further enhance your fitness level, keep yourself challenged and motivated, and integrate activity into your daily life.

The core mind/spirit program is established now, too. You're doing the 5-minute breather and practicing mindfulness throughout the day. You've established a bedtime ritual for yourself and are managing your time by turning down things you don't need to or don't have to do—and you're including more fun, enjoyable activities in your life. You'll continue to practice these skills for the remainder of the program, but from this point on, the "Feeling Good" elements are optional. Let me explain why. My intent is to make this a doable, manageable program you can keep up no matter how crazy your life gets—not to overwhelm you with additional responsibilities. If you'd like to try all six action steps in the "Feeling Good" section over the next six weeks, that's great—but if you'd prefer to only implement several, that's fine, too. My hope is that you'll choose at least three that you think you'll get the most benefit from. If you'd like to simplify your life, tackling a clutter-clearing project next week may be the impetus you need to get started; or if you haven't spent much quality time with your mate, Week 9's "Feeling Good" action step may give you the perfect excuse to plan a special date out.

So, how are you doing? How do you feel? Are you happier with the changes you've made? What additional improvements would you like to make? Take this opportunity to take a look at your *Food and Exercise Journal* and review your progress. Are you pleased with your accomplishments, or do you see that you've slacked off on some of the components of the program and need to recommit to it?

Let me emphasize that you don't have to have been "perfect" to have succeeded so far. What's important isn't perfection, but what I call "stick-to-it-ive-ness." That means when you miss a walk or eat too much at a meal, you don't give up—you simply continue on with the program. Forget the "all or nothing" mindset—in real life, and in this program, you simply do the best you can. And if that's not perfect, that's fine.

If you're having trouble staying motivated, try these suggestions:

- Reread your "Dear Me" letter to remind yourself of why you want to make changes in your life.
- Read through your *Food and Exercise Journal* to discover how far you've come.
- Make a list of the changes you've seen since you started six weeks ago. Do you have more energy? Are your clothes looser? Do you feel less anxious? Carry these with you to remind you of your progress.
- Talk to your partner or a close friend. Ask for support—can he or she check in with you regularly to see how you're progressing?
- Treat yourself to something special for making it this far—and make the treat non–food related: maybe a new shirt, a new CD, or a massage. Hitting the halfway point deserves some celebrating!

your backup plan

If you've completely fallen by the wayside, though, you may need more than simply a quick review of your "Dear Me" letter. Maybe you've gotten sick and have been barely able to leave your bed, much less walk 3 times a week. Or you've faced a family crisis or been traveling and found it impossible to eat as healthfully as you want. Now you're short on motivation and long on guilt, and you're tempted to throw in the towel because even this 12-Week Action Plan seems overwhelming.

Before you give up, recognize that setbacks are inevitable. Everyone has them. But what sets apart those people who succeed at changing their lives is that instead of getting derailed by setbacks, they implement a backup plan. You should do the same.

If you've been unable to exercise 3 times a week, for example, your "Plan B" might be to exercise once a week—or to simply get up more often at work to walk around. Can't make all the dietary changes? Focus instead on one or two—like drinking more water, eating more fruits and vegetables, or paying attention to your portion size. Instead of focusing on all the things you're *not* doing, focus on what you *can* do—and don't beat yourself up because you've "failed."

One of the best ways to stay on track regardless of obstacles is to let go of blame and give yourself credit for what you are doing. Feeling guilty doesn't get you anywhere. I know it can be tough to change habits that may have been ingrained for years, and some people have an easier time changing their lifestyles than others do. But if you can continue to focus on *small* changes, you will still continue to improve your health. Be patient and don't jump back into the program full strength until you're ready to do so. Remember, even the smallest of changes adds up to big results.

THIS WEEK'S CHANGES:

1. **Start reading the ingredient list on food labels.**

2. **Add core exercises to your workout.**

3. **Tackle a clutter-clearing project** (optional).

WEEK

7

EATING WELL
subtracting additives

So many products in the supermarket boast that they're "free" of something—fat-free, cholesterol-free, wheat-free, sugar-free, dairy-free, even guilt-free—that we tend to overlook a critical question: What is in it? In many products, you'd be hard-pressed to find a single ingredient remotely resembling something grown on a farm. We buy nonfat, sugar-free dessert topping because we're looking for a healthier alternative to whipped cream. But what is that fluffy white stuff anyway? Where does it come from? It may be nothing but a chemical cocktail, born in a laboratory. The bottom line may be that we're better off with the real version of whipped cream, saturated fat and all.

Companies use additives and chemically processed ingredients to make food more visually appealing, more flavorful, or more convenient. Most of these ingredients are safe. In fact, some even enhance the nutritional quality of our food. But many contribute to poor nutrition and are potentially dangerous. Two major additives, salt and sugar, are neither laboratory creations nor inherently bad, but have become a problem because they are used excessively. Other chemical additives have been proven safe in certain amounts but are questionable when used heavily. Still others have not been thoroughly tested and are possibly dangerous. Learning about how these ingredients may affect you will help you choose your food more wisely.

Modern technology has given us safer, more nutritious, and more convenient foods. But it has also laden our food supply with empty calories and potentially harmful chemicals. The trick is to be able to make the best choices in a marketplace that introduces thousands of new foods every year. This week, we're going to turn our attention to what is in our food besides the food itself, and make a habit of reading food labels to make educated decisions about what we buy at the grocery store.

how **overly** sweet it is

Americans have developed a huge sweet tooth. Every one of us consumes, on average, a shocking 150 pounds of refined sugar a year. Besides being a main ingredient in soda, candy, and sweet baked goods, sugar is packed into many "healthy" foods like cereals and dairy products. Our quest for fat-free cakes and cookies has not helped. Many fat-free confections have so much added sugar they wind up with the same number of calories as the full-fat variety. Sugar not only adds empty calories, which contribute to obesity and poor nutrition, but it also causes a rise in blood sugar that can, over time, contribute to heart disease and diabetes in some people.

Let's get one thing straight from the get-go: when I talk about sugar, I'm referring to added sugar—the sugar used to sweeten food—not the naturally occurring sugars inherent in food, like those in fruit (fructose) or integral to milk products (lactose). Our bodies process naturally occurring sugar and refined sugar the same way—both contain the same number of calories and cause a similar rise in blood sugar. But naturally occurring sugar is present in many foods that are essential for a healthy diet, such as fruits and dairy products. These foods are loaded with important vitamins, minerals, fiber, and phytonutrients that our bodies need.

By the way, I don't think added sugar is the devil in disguise. If it takes a sprinkle of brown sugar to get you to enjoy your oatmeal, go ahead and enjoy. A sprinkle here and there isn't a big deal. The problem is that so much sugar is added to food, it is hard to avoid it. So do yourself a favor and cut back on the stuff. Try to keep your added sugar intake to about 10 teaspoons (40 grams) a day—the amount of sugar in a single can of soda.

It's difficult to quantify the amount of added sugar in a product because food labels don't distinguish between sugars added in processing and those naturally occurring in the food. That means the label of *100 percent fruit juice* might list sugar content similar to that of a can of soda. But they are certainly not the same, nutritionally.

The best way to determine how much sugar is added to a food is to look at the ingredient list. On the label, ingredients are listed in order of quantity, from most to least. So if sugar and/or one of its many aliases—high-fructose corn syrup, fructose, invert sugar, dextrose, glucose, corn sugar, cane sugar, and corn syrup—is one of the first ingredients in your cereal, you may want to pick a different box. When you start reading labels, you may be amazed at how many products have several sources of sugar as their primary ingredients!

sweet alternatives

If you think swapping out your white granulated sugar bowl for a less-refined sugar like honey, raw sugar, brown sugar, maple syrup, or molasses is the answer, I have to tell you it's not. These choices are a notch better, and some provide minerals (molasses contains iron, magnesium, potassium, and calcium, for example), but the amounts are so small that it doesn't make much of a difference.

Artificial sweeteners offer sweetness without empty calories or blood-sugar effect, but be careful not to overdo them, either. Even the safest ones, aspartame (Nutra-Sweet, Equal) and sucralose (Splenda), are not necessarily safe in excessive amounts. Saccharin (Sweet 'N Low) should be avoided since it has been linked with cancer. Acesulfame-K (Sunett) is billed as safe, but many experts believe it has not been properly tested. Other sweeteners like mannitol and sorbitol, which are in many chewing gums and low-calorie foods, can, in large amounts, cause gastrointestinal upset and diarrhea.

When it comes to sweeteners (and most other things, actually), I believe *a little* of the real thing, in as unrefined form as possible, is the best way to go—unless, of course, you have a medical reason to avoid it. I am always a little suspicious of chemicals in my food, especially more recently developed ones. Even if current studies show they are benign, you never know how they will fare in the long term.

a grain of salt

There is a saying that the difference between a three-star restaurant and a four-star restaurant is a box of salt. Salt certainly makes food taste better. The problem is we eat too much of it. Most of us eat more than 4,000 milligrams a day, when the current guideline from the National Academy of Sciences Food and Nutrition Board is 1,500 milligrams. That's not surprising, considering a typical frozen dinner can have upward of 1,000 milligrams of sodium, and a half cup of canned soup can have more than 800 milligrams.

The issue of whether salt (and other sources of sodium) is linked to health problems has been hotly debated over the years. However, the latest research shows that high-sodium diets do lead to higher blood pressure. Most people's blood pressure inches up a little when they increase the salt in their diets, but those who are "salt-sensitive" experience dramatic blood pressure increases. Also, excessive sodium intake can cause calcium loss, which can weaken bones and contribute to osteoporosis.

Cutting back on salt doesn't mean you have to toss out the salt shaker or deprive yourself of flavor. Only 25 percent of the salt we eat comes from salt we add to food. Seventy-five percent comes from processed convenience foods and from dining out (at four-star restaurants and fast-food joints alike). Prepare your own meals from fresh, unprocessed food whenever possible (as you've been doing from Week 1!) and you'll automatically reduce your salt intake. Make sure to take advantage of lots of different flavorings—pepper, flavored vinegars, citrus juices, chili peppers, garlic, onions, and fresh herbs—to lessen your reliance on salt. Also read labels to find brands of canned, frozen, and packaged foods that are lower in sodium. There are a variety of low-sodium foods that are healthier and just as tasty.

the worst fat

As I explained in Week 5, the worst kind of fat for your health happens to be in just about every packaged baked good on the market, in many margarines and shortenings, and in many cereals and convenience foods. It is called trans fat. And, you'll recall it has the most dramatic effect on your heart of all the fats—potentially worse even than saturated fat.

Until 2006, when it becomes mandatory for companies to list trans fat on food labels, you may need to do a little detective work to determine how much of the fat is in a particular food. If trans fat isn't listed on the label's Nutrition Facts panel, there are two ways to detect it. First, you can deduce the grams of trans fat by adding up the grams of saturated, polyunsaturated, and monounsaturated fats and subtracting that number from the total fat. The difference is the amount of trans fat the food contains. Second, you can spot trans fat by looking for "hydrogenated or partially hydrogenated vegetable oil" on the ingredient list. If those ingredients are near the top, drop the box and run the other way. Then look for a similar product that is lower in total fat and/or says *trans-free* on the package. More manufacturers are making trans-free products now. But if you can't find what you are looking for in your regular grocery store, check out a health-food or whole-foods store.

go organic

Foods that carry the "USDA Certified Organic" label are grown without synthetic pesticides, raised without growth hormones or antibiotics, and farmed using sustainable, earth-friendly methods. While organic foods do not necessarily contain more nutrients than conventionally grown foods, they have fewer pesticide residues and are better for the environment. Also, many organic convenience foods are lower in additives, sugar, and sodium than their conventional counterparts. Organic foods may be more expensive, but if your budget allows it, I think the benefits are well worth the cost.

additives to avoid

Acesulfame potassium

Artificial sweetener found in baked goods, chewing gum, gelatin desserts, and soft drinks. Not adequately tested. Linked with various diseases.

Artificial colorings
    Blue 1, Blue 2,
    Green 3, Red 3,
    Yellow 3

Found in beverages, candy, and baked goods. May cause hyperactivity in sensitive children. Studies show possible links with cancer.

Cyclamate

Artificial sweetener found in diet foods. Linked with cancer.

Olestra

Fat substitute found in chips and crackers. Can cause diarrhea, loose stools, abdominal cramps, and flatulence. Reduces body's ability to absorb fat-soluble nutrients.

Potassium Bromate

Flour improver found in bread and rolls. May cause cancer.

Propyl Gallate

Preservative used in vegetable oil, meat products, potato sticks, chicken soup base, chewing gum. Some studies suggest a link with cancer.

Saccharin

Artificial sweetener in diet products, soft drinks, and packets. Causes cancer in animals.

Sodium nitrite, sodium nitrate

Preservatives and coloring agents used in cured meats and fish (bacon, ham, frank-furters, smoked fish). Several studies show a link with cancer.

Copyright 2004 CSPI. Reprinted/Adapted from *Nutrition Action Healthletter.*

other additives

And then there are the other additives—emulsifiers, thickeners, stabilizers, preservatives, chelating agents, artificial flavorings, artificial colorings . . . all with such mind-boggling names that if I printed them here, your head would spin. Most of them are safe, however. Some are actually essential nutrients put to good use: alpha-tocopherol (vitamin E) is used as a preservative, and ascorbic acid (vitamin C) is used as a color stabilizer, for example. Others are potentially harmful. The Center for Science in the Public Interest, a consumer watchdog group, puts out a list of additives to avoid, which I have summarized in the box opposite. There is evidence that these additives are unsafe in the amounts they are commonly used, or they are very poorly tested.

recipe

macaroni and cheese SERVES 8

This kid-friendly macaroni and cheese gets its bright orange color from nutrient-packed winter squash, not artificial dyes.

Cooking spray

1 pound elbow macaroni

2 12-ounce packages of frozen cooked
   winter squash (about 2^1/$_2$ cups)

2 cups nonfat milk

4 ounces extra-sharp cheddar cheese,
   grated (about 1^1/$_4$ cup)

^{1}/$_2$ cup part-skim ricotta cheese

^{1}/$_2$ teaspoon salt

1 teaspoon powdered mustard

^{1}/$_8$ teaspoon cayenne pepper

2 tablespoons grated Parmesan cheese

2 tablespoons unseasoned bread crumbs

1 teaspoon canola oil

Preheat oven to 375°F. Coat a 9-by-13-inch baking pan with cooking spray.

Bring a large pot of water to a boil. Add the macaroni and cook until tender but firm, about 5–8 minutes. Drain and transfer to a large bowl.

Meanwhile, place frozen squash in a large saucepan and defrost over a low flame, stirring occasionally. Add the milk and turn the heat up to medium. Cook until almost boiling, stirring occasionally. Remove from heat and stir in cheddar cheese, ricotta cheese, salt, mustard, and cayenne pepper. Pour cheese mixture over macaroni and stir to combine. Transfer the macaroni and cheese to the baking dish.

Combine bread crumbs, Parmesan cheese, and oil in a small bowl. Sprinkle over the top of the macaroni and cheese. Bake for 30 minutes. Then broil for 3 minutes so the top is crisp and nicely browned.

Calories 357; Fat 8 g (Sat 4.3 g, Mono 2.3 g, Poly .8 g); Protein 16.3 g; Carb 55.2 g; Fiber 1.4 g; Chol 22 mg; Sodium 328 mg

ACTION

Your action this week is to start reading food labels. Focus mainly on the ingredient list to see what the food is made of. Before buying a product, scan the ingredients for sugars, trans fats, and additives to avoid; also check the sodium content. Then decide if this is something you want to put in your body or if there is a better alternative. The good news is that by following the "Usually/Sometimes/Rarely" list, you have already given a backseat to most unhealthy foods.

GETTING FIT
strengthening your core

This week, you'll learn about your "core" and why keeping it strong and flexible is one of the best ways to maintain your overall fitness—and prevent common injuries as well.

your core and what it does

First things first: what is your *core,* anyway? It's basically another word for your torso, and includes the muscles of your abdomen and back. While you may not be aware of it, your core is an essential part of every motion you make. It stabilizes you while you sit, stand, walk, and move and affects your balance and posture.

Until recently, many people didn't pay much attention to their core other than doing the typical sit-ups, crunches, or other exercises designed to flatten their stomachs. Now, however, fitness professionals are discovering the importance of strengthening the core muscles and dedicate whole classes to focusing on this area. Disciplines like yoga and Pilates also target the core muscles.

Fitness experts say that exercising your core can help strengthen and even lengthen your spine, improve your balance and circulation, and help streamline your body. Core training should be an essential part of your regular fitness routine, and in fact it's considered "functional" exercise—meaning that it helps enhance your daily activities. A strong, flexible core is the centerpiece of a fit, healthy body.

stronger core, better posture

A strong core also helps you maintain proper posture—and vice versa. Simply walking with proper posture strengthens your core muscles, and good posture makes you look taller and trimmer, as well as reducing your risk of injury. Proper posture involves a "neutral" spine, where you have a slight curve in your lower back that gives you flexibility and helps protect your back. Your stomach should be tucked in, your head up. If your core is weak, however, you may tend to slump forward at

pilates

Chances are you've heard of Pilates (puh-la-teez) by now—in fact, your local gym may offer classes in it. Pilates has grown increasingly popular over the past decade, in part because of celebrities who swear by it. This discipline can help you develop a core that not only looks great but is stronger and more flexible as well.

Joseph Pilates, a personal trainer from Germany, developed Pilates in the 1920s. He drew on martial arts, Eastern philosophies, and physical training methods to create a series of exercises that focus on balancing muscular strength, increasing flexibility, and providing total body awareness.

Pilates moves center around your core, also referred to as the *powerhouse,* the area between your rib cage and your pelvis that includes your abdominal and gluteus muscles. Because most Pilates exercises involve few repetitions and slow, controlled movements, you may find it a relaxing change of pace from higher-intensity workouts.

Just as there are different types and styles of yoga, there are different versions of Pilates, too. There's traditional Pilates (or Pilates, Inc.), Stott Pilates, Polestar Pilates, the Method Pilates (also known as Physical Mind Pilates), and others. While each is based on Pilates's principles of flowing motion and fluidity and use the same basic moves, different versions vary in terms of their emphasis—Stott Pilates, for example, aims to restore the natural curves of the spine, while traditional Pilates focuses more on flattening the spine.

the shoulders. Check your posture several times a day—you don't have to sit and stand ramrod straight, but we tend to slump as we tire.

As people grow older, their posture also tends to worsen—weakened muscles and even bone loss contribute to poor posture. But the strengthening and stretching moves you learned in the previous weeks and the core exercises you'll start doing this week will help give you better posture now and in the years to come. While these moves target your core, you can work this area during any type of exercise. For example, if you're walking or jogging, make sure you're maintaining good posture. During strength training, your movements should involve your core: for example, while doing pushups, focus on keeping your abdominal muscles tight; when you do squats, maintain good posture with your head up, shoulders back, and tummy tucked in. Even simple movements like balancing on one leg for a few minutes will strengthen your core muscles.

four for the core

Simply by focusing on good posture no matter what you're doing, you strengthen and tone your core muscles. Exercises that involve balance also target your core because your body uses these muscles to stabilize itself. For example, stability balls are now popular for training your core because you must balance on the ball while performing exercises.

Simply being aware of your core will improve your posture and balance, but these exercises specifically target your core muscles to strengthen them and help prevent injuries. Proper form is important, so focus on doing the moves in a slow, controlled fashion while keeping your torso stable.

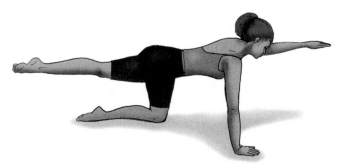

Pointer dog
On all fours, lift up your right arm and your left leg at the same time, extend them out, and hold for three breaths. Switch to the other side (left arm and right leg).

Side plank

Lie on your left side, with bent legs stacked and your weight on your left forearm, elbow directly under your shoulder. Raise your hips off the floor, straighten your top leg, and hold for three breaths (or until you become tired)—your body should be a straight line between your elbow and knee. Then roll to your right side and repeat.

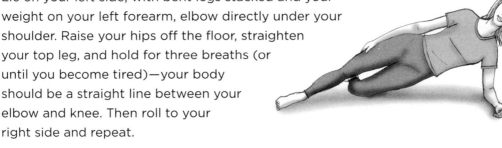

Back bridge

Lie on the floor with your knees bent, feet flat on the floor, arms at your sides. Lift your hips and lower back to form a straight line from your knees to your chest, and hold for three breaths. (As you become stronger, you can extend one foot at a time to make the move more difficult.)

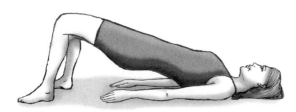

One-leg balancer

Stand up, your legs shoulder-distance apart, your head lifted, shoulders back. With your arms at your sides or outstretched for balance, lift one foot off the floor, keeping your leg straight, and hold it up while balancing on your other leg. (It may be harder than you think!) Hold for three breaths and repeat on the other side. (If you worry about falling, do this move next to a wall for support.)

beat back injuries

Chances are that at some point, you'll hurt your back—more than 80 percent of Americans will experience back pain at least once in their lives. Fortunately, most back pain can be alleviated with rest, stretches, exercises, and drugs to relieve pain and reduce inflammation. While minor injuries should heal quickly, preventive medicine can help forestall an injury from occurring before it happens.

Back injuries are common because of the way our bodies are designed. Our backs have supporting ligaments and muscles that allow us to stand up straight while allowing flexibility. However, this flexibility also creates the risk of injuring the muscles, ligaments, and other soft tissue that support the spine. If you don't keep these supporting muscles and ligaments strong, you're more likely to hurt your back—that's why core strength is so important. Reduce your risk of a back injury by following these tips:

MAINTAIN GOOD POSTURE If you sit at work, use a chair with a strong back and sit as far back in your seat as possible. Get up and take short walking breaks whenever you can.

START OFF SLOWLY It's ironic that some back injuries are caused by working out. So ease into a workout routine slowly.

STRETCH IT OUT Stretching helps maintain your overall flexibility and prevent muscular stiffness that can throw your back out of balance.

STAY TRIM Maintaining a healthy weight will reduce your risk of injuries—carrying extra poundage, especially around your waist, ups the chance of back pain.

ACTION

Add the core training moves to your workout 3 times this week.

clearing clutter

the clutter crisis

Be honest: How does your house look? What's the state of your desk at work? Is it organized and comfortable? Does it take you only a moment to find anything you need—or do you spend 10 minutes every day searching for your keys? If you've been overcome by clutter, there are some practical ways to help get things back under control.

One of the tenets of feng shui, an ancient Chinese philosophy of nature, is to eliminate unused objects and possessions to create clear spaces in your environment. The idea is that these clear spaces also create space in your mind and in your life for the things you want, and help reduce stress. Eliminating clutter can not only make your home seem larger, it can also make you feel calmer and more relaxed.

What is clutter? Anything you own that you no longer use, need, or love. It's everything from unread magazines to clothes that don't fit anymore to gifts you received but feel guilty about throwing out. And most of our homes are filled with it.

Getting rid of clutter is easier than you might think. First, decide it's time to streamline your life, and then start out slowly. You'll probably find that it gets easier as you go along—your home is less crowded, your life feels more manageable, and you can finally locate your keys!

Here's a simple process to help you sort the "keepers" from the clutter in your life:

1. Ask yourself, "Do I really need this [dress/book/CD/trinket/end table/fill in the blank]? Do I love it? Do I use it/read it/wear it/listen to it? If I didn't have it, would I miss it tomorrow? Will I ever use it again?" If the answers to these questions are no, it's clutter.

2. Put it in a box You can donate these items to charity, give them to a friend, recycle them, or sell them at a garage sale. But physically remove them from the rest of your stuff—and get them out of your home as soon as possible. Otherwise, those objects tend to migrate back into your home.

3. Go step by step You can't declutter your entire home in a weekend. You can start off small—your desk or underwear drawer, for example—and go from there. Build your momentum with smaller jobs before you tackle the garage, basement, or attic.

4. Cut yourself some slack I'm not saying you must toss your daughter's baby blanket or any other object that holds special meaning to you. If your heart breaks at the thought of losing something, keep it. But if it's a sweater that you detest, why not lighten your load and get rid of it? Donating things you don't want and need to people who can use them is the best way to get over any residual "gift-getting guilt"—that feeling you get when you receive a present you can't stand, yet feel bad about disposing of.

ACTION

This week's optional action is simple: tackle one "clearing clutter" project. Choose an area of your home that needs it—whether the junk drawer in your kitchen or your linen closet—and give yourself 30 minutes to do as much as you can. You'll be amazed at how much progress you can make in a short time.

action summary

EATING WELL
- Shop to replenish your healthy pantry.
- Eat regular meals and snacks, stopping when you are at a 5 or 6 on the hunger scale.
- Drink enough to stay well hydrated, including at least five glasses of water and a maximum of one sugary drink a day.
- Use healthy fats for cooking, dressings, and spreads.
- Eat two to four servings of fruit and three to six servings of vegetables each day.
- Check the ingredient list on your food labels.
- Record in your journal everything you eat and drink.

GETTING FIT
- Walk for 20 to 30 minutes 3 times at mid-intensity.
- Stretch and do strength training and core training 3 times.
- Include a fun element in your fitness program.
- Note your activity in your journal.

FEELING GOOD
- Do the 5-minute breather or mini-vacation once a day.
- Practice mindfulness.
- Say "no" to tasks you don't want to and don't have to do.
- Keep up your bedtime ritual.
- Do a deep-relaxation or meditation exercise at least once this week.
- Optional: tackle a clutter-clearing project.

WEIGHT _____

THIS WEEK'S CHANGES:

1. Go for whole grains and limit refined grains.

2. Sign up for a fitness class.

3. Explore journaling (optional).

WEEK 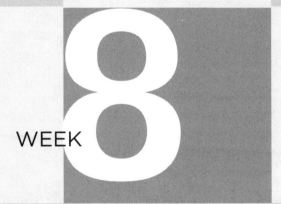**8**

go with the grain

Not too long ago carbohydrates were the "chosen" foods. Dieters and athletes alike would eat bagels and pasta all day, often to the exclusion of most other foods. It was all part of the fat-free craze I was talking about in Week 7. Now the diet pendulum has swung the other way, and it is all the rage to cut carbs completely out of your diet.

Guess what. Neither extreme works. As usual, you need to find the proper balance—and I'm going to help you do just that.

Remember that all of our caloric needs come from three sources—carbohydrates, protein, and fat. For the record, carbohydrate is the component of food that supplies the body with its most readily available source of energy. That's because it breaks down quickly to become glucose, the body's main energy currency.

Carbohydrates are divided into two types: simple and complex. Simple carbohydrates are sugars that include refined white sugar, maple syrup, honey, corn syrup, and molasses as well as the sugar in fruits, vegetables, and dairy products. Complex carbohydrates are starches found primarily in grains like rice, wheat, and barley, and in "starchy" vegetables like potatoes and corn. While fruits and vegetables are comprised mostly of carbohydrates, when people talk about "carbs" they usually mean the starchy ones found in bread, rice, potatoes, and pasta. This week we're going to focus primarily on this group of carbs, and how to incorporate the right *amount* and the right *kinds* of grains and other starches into your diet.

separating the wheat from the chaff

You see it on *Entertainment Tonight,* and on the cover of *People* magazine—all the celebrities are cutting carbs to keep in shape. These days, a carb-free diet is the fashionable thing to follow. It certainly seems enticing—stop eating bread, look like Jennifer Aniston. Too bad it doesn't work that way. Sure, most people would be a lot trimmer if they cut back on—or eliminated—*certain* carbohydrate-rich foods from their diets. But there is absolutely no reason to go the rest of your life without eating a sandwich or a dish of pasta.

For most of us, the problem isn't eating carbs per se, but eating too much of the wrong kind of carbs. White breads, heavily sweetened cereals, cakes, doughnuts, cookies, and snack foods (most of which are also sugary and fatty) are easy to overeat and don't offer much in terms of nutrition. So if eating fewer carbs means you're no

keeping tabs on blood sugar

It used to be that only people with diabetes thought about watching their blood sugar, but there is mounting evidence that keeping blood sugar in check, even if you are healthy, may prevent chronic disease and help you manage your weight. Carbohydrate-rich foods have the biggest impact on blood sugar, but some cause a much steeper spike than others. How much of an effect a food has on blood sugar depends on a number of factors including how much fat, protein, and fiber the food contains; the manner in which it is prepared; and of course the amount you eat.

You may have heard of the Glycemic Index (GI), a commonly seen measure of how different carbohydrate foods affect blood sugar. While the GI can be useful, one problem is that it compares an amount of a food containing a set amount of carbohydrate (50 grams) against a standard, without regard for typical portion sizes. For example, carrots have a fairly high GI, but you would have to eat seven whole carrots to get 50 grams' worth of carbohydrate! So the GI doesn't always reflect how the food is eaten in the real world. A new measure called the Glycemic Load (GL) is based on the GI but is even more useful because it takes portion sizes into account when ranking foods—and as a result, carrots have a low GL.

If you look at the list on page 151, you'll see that the foods with the lower GL are generally the least processed and the most nutritious—vegetables, whole fruits, whole grains, and beans. One notable exception—potatoes, which are extremely nutritious—also have a very high GL.

When choosing which carbohydrates to eat, take the GL into consideration, but don't forget the big picture. It is generally a good idea to focus on foods with a low GL, but it is also important to factor in the nutritional value of the food, and the other foods you're consuming with it. GL reflects the blood-sugar effect of a single item, but that effect is buffered in the context of a meal.

The bottom line: to keep blood sugar in line, eat whole, unprocessed grains, fruits, and vegetables; avoid foods with added sugar; keep portions small; and eat some protein and/or healthy fat along with the carbohydrate in your meal or snack.

longer snarfing the whole basket of rolls at dinner, eating piles of mashed potatoes, and munching on corn chips, great. But please, don't cut grains and starchy vegetables completely out of your diet. If you do, you'll be missing out on some of the most nutritious, satisfying foods available—foods that most of us need to eat *more,* not less, of.

the whole story

Let me tell you the life story of a grain. Every grain (like wheat, rice, barley, oats, and the like) is born with three parts—endosperm, bran, and germ. Intact, each grain is loaded with fiber, minerals like copper, zinc, and magnesium, essential B vitamins, vitamin E, disease-fighting phytonutrients, and even some protein. It is a proud and hearty little nugget of nourishment.

Then comes a big turning point in the grain's life. It's harvested and taken to the mill, where its bran and germ are removed and its endosperm, which is mostly starch, is ground into flour. Since most of the grain's nutritional power is found in the bran and germ, the milled (refined) flour offers little besides calories. To make up for this loss, manufacturers "enrich" the flour with vitamins and minerals. The enrichment process helps return some potency to the grain, but even then it is a shadow of its former self. It can never regain the wealth of health benefits it once had. Sad, isn't it? Forget "Save the whales." I say, "Save the grains!"

Seriously, though, whole grains with the bran, endosperm, and germ intact have some remarkable health benefits. More than twenty-five studies have proven that people who regularly eat whole grains have a lower risk of heart disease than those who do not. One study showed a 30 percent reduction in one type of heart disease in postmenopausal women who ate at least one serving of whole grain a day. More than forty different studies examining twenty types of cancer have found that regularly eating whole grains can reduce cancer risk by 10 percent to 60 percent, depending on the type of cancer. Whole grains also have a lower glycemic load (see Keeping Tabs on Blood Sugar, page 148) than refined grains, so they don't cause the rapid rise in blood sugar and insulin (a hormone that controls blood sugar), which can contribute to diabetes and other health problems.

getting more whole grains

While you may not have known *all* the wonders of whole grains, chances are I'm not telling you anything entirely new. Ninety percent of Americans believe that whole-grain breads and cereals are healthier than "regular" products. Yet we're not eating them like we should. Two thirds of us don't even get a single daily serving of whole grains, while ideally you want to have at least three servings per day.

This is easier than it sounds. Simply switching to 100 percent whole wheat bread, and starting your day with a whole-grain cereal like Cheerios, Shredded Wheat, Raisin Bran, or oatmeal, will easily put you in the recommended range of three daily servings. To take it a step further, serve brown rice at dinner, make whole wheat pasta, try whole wheat couscous, and explore exotic grains like bulgur and quinoa (keen-wah). Choose corn tortillas and snack on baked corn chips or low-fat popcorn—all are whole grain. Get a jar of wheat germ to sprinkle on yogurt and salad or put it in pancake and muffin batter and smoothies. Wheat germ is loaded with minerals, vitamins (it is one of the best sources of vitamin E), and fiber. Not to mention that it adds a wonderful texture and flavor to foods.

Ever the realist, I am not saying you have to eat only whole grains (but, by all means, go ahead, if you'd like). I personally prefer regular pasta in most recipes, enjoy both brown rice and white rice, and sometimes I simply must have a bit of crusty French bread. What I am asking you to do is to choose whole grains whenever possible, to make them one of your "Usually" foods.

savvy shopping

When you are choosing whole-grain products, you have to be a savvy shopper because many foods that look like whole grain are not. I'd like to clear up a big source of confusion right now: *wheat* bread does not necessarily mean *whole wheat* bread—it just means bread that's made of wheat. People and manufacturers often use those terms interchangeably, and it is confusing. Also, just because a bread is brown and has flecks of fiber in it doesn't mean it is whole grain. Sometimes manufacturers add brown coloring and bits of fiber to make bread *appear* more wholesome. The word *multigrain* is also misleading: it doesn't mean the grains are whole, but just that there is more than one type of grain in the product.

The best way to tell if a product is whole grain is to check the ingredient list on the label. Ideally, you should find the words *100% whole wheat,* or *100% whole grain;* at the minimum, whole wheat or whole grain should be one of the first ingredients.

pass the potatoes . . . and the corn

While corn and potatoes are vegetables, because they are starchy vegetables, I consider them as part of this grain group for nutritional purposes. What you really need to know is that they are good for you.

Potatoes are, I think, an unfairly maligned food. White potatoes are rich in vitamin C, potassium, fiber, and minerals, and they are deliciously satisfying. Yes, they can cause a rapid rise in blood sugar. But that is tempered when they are eaten—as they usually are—as part of a meal containing protein and some fat. I believe that for most people, the nutritional benefits of potatoes far outweigh their detrimental blood-sugar effects. Unless you have a known problem with your blood sugar, go ahead and enjoy potatoes.

Sweet potatoes are also an excellent starch choice, and one of the best sources of beta-carotene available. I always bake a few extras so I have them on hand for a quick snack—they're delicious served cold with a scoop of cottage cheese and sprinkled cinnamon on top.

Corn is also a starchy vegetable that includes a wealth of nutrients. It is often used as a grain, and foods made of ground corn, like corn tortillas, are considered to be whole grain. Opting for corn tortillas over white-flour ones is an easy way to up your whole-grain intake.

FOOD	GLYCEMIC LOAD (GL)
Carrots	3
Chickpeas	3
Popcorn	4
Orange, whole	5
Whole-grain bread	7
All-Bran cereal	9
White bread	10
Banana	13
Spaghetti	15
Coca-Cola	16
Corn Flakes	24
Bagel	25
Baked potato	26

don't fill up on bread

Even now, I can hear my grandmother's admonition as clear as day—"Don't fill up on bread." As usual, Grandma was right. Even if the bread is whole grain, it's not a good idea to eat the whole loaf. The main reason people gain weight from grains and starches is that they just plain overeat them. I have six words for you, folks: portion control, portion control, portion control.

Whatever kind of grain or starchy vegetable you choose, I recommend keeping your servings to between four and nine a day, depending on your calorie range found on page 237. That may sound like a lot, but those servings are smaller than you might think: one serving is 1 slice of bread; $^1/_2$ cup cooked grain, pasta, or cereal; $^3/_4$ cup cold ready-to-eat cereal; $^1/_2$ pita pocket; one medium potato; or 1 ear of corn. Next time you go to a restaurant, notice that a bowl of pasta is about 2 cups—that's 4 servings right there! And a New York–style bagel is the equivalent of 4 slices of bread. With servings like that, it is easy to overeat if you're not careful.

recipes

whole wheat penne with sausage and broccoli rabe SERVES 4

The rich flavors of sausage and broccoli rabe stand up well to the nutty taste of the whole wheat pasta. Broccoli rabe is one of my favorite vegetables, but it has a bitter taste that isn't for everyone. Feel free to substitute regular broccoli in this recipe.

1 bunch broccoli rabe (about 1 pound), washed and coarsely chopped
$^1/_4$ cup pine nuts
$^3/_4$ pound whole wheat penne
2 tablespoons olive oil
$^3/_4$ pound low-fat Italian-style poultry sausage

3 garlic cloves, minced
1 cup low-sodium chicken broth
$^1/_4$ teaspoon crushed red pepper flakes
Salt and freshly ground black pepper to taste
$^1/_4$ cup grated Parmesan cheese

Preheat the oven to 350°F.

Place the broccoli rabe in a large microwaveable dish with 1 tablespoon of water. Cover tightly and microwave on high for 5 minutes. Drain and set aside.

Spread the pine nuts in a single layer on a baking sheet and toast in the oven for about 5 minutes, or until they are fragrant and golden brown.

Set a large pot of water to boil for the pasta. When boiling, add the pasta and cook according to the directions on the box, about 12 minutes. Drain.

Meanwhile, heat 1 tablespoon of the oil in a large skillet over a medium flame. Add the sausage and cook for 5 or 6 minutes, until brown. Remove the sausage from the skillet and slice into rounds.

Add the remaining oil to the skillet and sauté the garlic until fragrant, about 2 minutes. Stir in the broccoli rabe and sliced sausage and sauté for about 3 minutes. Add the chicken broth, crushed red pepper, and salt and pepper to taste. Simmer on a low heat until pasta is ready.

Combine the drained pasta with the sausage–broccoli rabe mixture and the pine nuts in a large bowl or pot. Serve topped with Parmesan cheese.

Calories 612; Fat 18.6 g (Sat 4.5 g, Mono 8.4 g, Poly 3.5 g); Protein 30 g; Carb 81.2 g; Fiber 5.9 g; Chol 43 mg; Sodium 885 mg

wild rice salad SERVES 8

Wild rice is a protein-rich whole grain that is native to North America. It has a delicious, nutty flavor.

$^3/_4$ cup wild rice

$^1/_4$ cup brown rice

1 cup chopped walnuts

$^3/_4$ cup dried cranberries

$^1/_2$ cup chopped fresh flat-leaf parsley

$^1/_4$ cup chopped scallion

2 tablespoons olive oil

2 tablespoons balsamic vinegar

1 teaspoon Dijon mustard

1 garlic clove, minced (optional)

Bring 2 cups of water to a boil in a medium saucepan with a tight-fitting lid. Stir in the wild rice and brown rice, reduce the heat to low, cover, and cook for 45 minutes, or until all the water is absorbed.

Preheat the oven to 400°F. Spread the walnuts in a single layer on a baking tray and toast for 5 minutes.

Transfer the cooked rices to a large mixing bowl. Stir in the toasted nuts, cranberries, parsley, and scallion.

In a medium bowl, whisk together the oil, vinegar, mustard, and garlic, if using. Pour over the rice mixture. Stir to combine; serve chilled.

Calories 216; Fat 13.5 g (Sat 1.4 g, Mono 3.9 g, Poly 7.5 g); Protein 5.2 g; Carb 20.6 g; Fiber 2.9 g; Chol 0 mg; Sodium 19 mg

tabbouleh SERVES 8

At first glance you might think this dish calls for too much parsley, but heaps of fresh parsley define this classic Middle Eastern whole-grain salad.

1 cup bulgur wheat

2 medium tomatoes, diced (about 2 cups)

1 cucumber, peeled, seeded, and diced (about 1½ cups)

½ cup diced red onion

2 cups finely chopped fresh flat-leaf parsley

⅓ cup finely chopped fresh mint leaves

3 tablespoons olive oil

¼ cup freshly squeezed lemon juice

Salt and freshly ground black pepper to taste

Cook the bulgur according to the directions on the package and let it cool. In a large bowl combine the bulgur with the tomatoes, cucumber, onion, parsley, and mint. Drizzle the olive oil and lemon juice on top and toss. Season with salt and pepper to taste. Cover and place in the refrigerator for 1 hour or more. Serve chilled.

Calories 128; Fat 5.6 g (Sat .8 g, Mono 3.8 g, Poly .6 g); Protein 3.3 g; Carb 18.4 g; Fiber 4.6 g; Chol 0 mg; Sodium 15 mg

baked fries SERVES 4

I have to confess that French fries are one of my favorite foods. These easy-to-make "fries" satisfy my cravings without all the unhealthy fat.

3 large baking potatoes, such as russets

1 tablespoon canola oil

Cooking spray

Salt to taste

Preheat the oven to 450°F.

Cut the potatoes lengthwise into 10 to 12 even-sized wedges. Place them in a large bowl and toss with the oil.

Spray a baking sheet with cooking spray and place the potatoes on the tray in a single layer. Bake for 20 minutes. Use a metal spatula to scrape the wedges from the pan and turn them over with a fork or tongs, keeping them in a single layer. Bake for 15 minutes longer, or until golden and crisp. Season with salt to taste.

Calories 171; Fat 3.6 g (Sat .3 g, Mono 2 g, Poly 1.1 g); Protein 3.8 g; Carb 32 g; Fiber 3.3 g; Chol 0 mg; Sodium 15 mg

ACTION

Your mission this week is to get at least three servings of whole grains a day, and keep your total servings of grains (bread, rice, pasta, crackers, etc.) and starchy vegetables (corn and potatoes) to between four and nine servings, depending on your calorie range. (See page 237.)

(See page 237.)

GETTING FIT

exercise your options

This week you'll learn how exercise classes can add variety and fun to your regular workout routine. Maybe you're already a fan, but even if you've never taken a class before or prefer to work out alone, group workouts can be a great way to add something new to the mix.

join the crowd!

Some people like to work out alone; others prefer to exercise with another person or a group. Even if you usually work out solo, an exercise class can breathe new life into your routine:

- **It adds a social aspect to your workout.** It's difficult enough to find the time and motivation to exercise. In a group, you don't have to go it alone—you're surrounded by like-minded people who are all there to get in shape and have fun. You can take a class with someone you already know, or make new friends by attending classes—sweating together is a great ice-breaker. Plus, after a good workout, people tend to be relaxed and friendly.
- **It forces you to make a commitment.** If exercise tends to be the last thing on your to-do list, signing up for a class can help keep you working out regularly. The class is already scheduled—all you have to do is show up. And since you've already paid for the class, you're more likely to attend.

(Exercising solo, you can always promise yourself you'll work out later . . . and then skip it.)

■ **It adds variety to your mix.** Most of us are creatures of habit. This may keep you exercising regularly, but you're bound to get bored doing the same workout day after day. Learning new skills challenges your body (and your mind) in new ways and forces you to use different muscle groups.

what's right for you?

So, which class is right for you? The answer will depend in part on your fitness level, workout goals, and personality. But don't automatically assume that just because you're low-key, you need to stick with slow-paced classes. Something different and higher energy like kickboxing or spinning may fit the bill.

Think about how you spend your day—a workout that's the *opposite* of that may be the most enjoyable for you. If you're on the go all day, a stretching or yoga class may be a great way to relax. If you have a desk job, though, you may want to choose something more active to get your blood pumping and leave behind workplace stressors.

Check out what your local gym, YMCA, or health club offers. Many community centers, colleges, and schools also offer inexpensive fitness classes for local resi-

take a lesson

You say a group class isn't quite your thing? Is your schedule too unpredictable to make attending regularly possible? If you can't exercise with a group, consider working out with a personal trainer or taking a lesson in a new sport or activity.

Lessons for adults are nothing new—a professional coach can give you tips to improve your golf swing or help you with your tennis serve. Working one-on-one with a pro can give you the skills and confidence you need to continue with a new sport.

In a similar way, a personal trainer can evaluate your fitness and your current workout program, modify it to address your fitness goals, and keep you motivated. Personal training and coaching sessions aren't just for the rich and famous—many gyms offer discounts for members, or you can sign up with a friend for a joint session to save money. They'll work around your schedule and may be well worth the investment.

dents. If you haven't taken an exercise class before, you may be amazed at the variety now available, including:

- **Dance such as ballet, hip-hop, tap, or modern** Most clubs offer dance classes for levels from beginners to advanced. Do you secretly wish you could groove like Beyoncé? Wanted to take ballet as a child but didn't? Here's your chance.
- **Couples dance** With a partner, you can learn how to swing dance, square dance, or master the steps of the rhumba. Ballroom and swing classes are popular with couples of all ages—it's a great way to spend time with your partner and enjoy yourself while you're getting fitter.
- **Spinning** This popular high-intensity class uses stationary bicycles for an intense cardio workout. Make sure to take a water bottle and a towel—you'll sweat!
- **Pilates classes** There are a variety of Pilates methods to choose from (see page 139); most focus on no-impact mat workouts that emphasize strength, flexibility, and proper breathing.
- **Body pump or group weight-training** Now you can weight train in a group setting: the instructor tells you which moves to perform, and you select the weight that's right for you. It's a fun way to strength train.
- **Stretching** These focus on increasing flexibility and are usually low key, a good way to decompress at the end of the day.
- **Tai chi** This traditional Chinese regimen involves slow, smooth, gentle movements that require the integration of the body and mind. It's appropriate for almost any level of fitness.
- **Yoga** Yoga focuses on flexibility, strength, and balance. Hatha yoga classes are usually the lowest intensity while other types are more difficult. (See Yoga: The All-Over Workout, page 158.)
- **Boot camp** The classes focus on basic athletic exercises and sports drills; they are usually fairly high intensity, but some are designed for beginners.
- **Tae bo or kickboxing** These classes incorporate self-defense techniques and drills to enhance your strength and endurance.
- **Step** You can get a high-intensity, low-impact aerobic workout with step classes. They've been around for twenty years but are still popular.
- **Aerobics** These range from basic, low-impact moves to high-intensity classes for the fittest; the movements may be simple or more complex.

yoga: the all-over workout

Seems like everybody's doing it these days. Yoga, that is.

This ancient Indian practice enhances flexibility, builds strength, and tones the body while focusing on mind-body unity. The word *yoga* means "to join," which refers to linking the mind and body. Yoga uses mental focus, breathing, and physical movements together to achieve this connection.

There are dozens of types and schools of yoga, some of which are fairly simple while others are more demanding. Yoga instills a sense of calm and relaxation, but it also boosts stamina as well. The focus on deep breathing helps distribute more oxygen throughout your body, which has both a calming and energizing effect. It also increases flexibility and range of motion.

Even if you've tried yoga before and weren't crazy about it, don't give up. Classes and instructors vary widely in their approach and the forms, or poses, they use. Some of the most popular forms of yoga include:

- **HATHA** While many forms of yoga fall under the basic category of hatha, generally this means yoga that uses the practice of *asanas,* or postures, to help balance, purify, and strengthen the body and that incorporates breath flow. Often hatha classes offered by gyms are aimed at beginners or people new to yoga.

- **BIKRAM** This yoga includes very demanding physical poses that are practiced in a heated room (usually about 105 degrees Fahrenheit) to allow muscles, ligaments, and joints to stretch further. It's demanding and not for beginners.

- **ASHTANGA** One type of ashtanga is what's called power yoga. In general, ashtanga is a faster paced, gymnastic-type yoga where a lot of emphasis is placed on challenging, energizing postures.

- **IYENGAR** This type puts more emphasis on form and less on breath control. It's very structured and puts a lot of attention on alignment.

tone up with tai chi

Yoga isn't the only Eastern art that has grown in popularity in recent years. Tai chi, tai kwando, kyudo kai (Japanese archery), and other arts are also popular.

Nearly anyone can do tai chi. Its slow, flowing movements are simple yet deceptively effective—studies have found that practicing tai chi reduces stress, improves balance and coordination, increases flexibility, motion, and strength, improves body awareness, burns calories, and assists in mental well-being.

Tai chi movements are performed in a low, nearly squatting position that helps strengthen the back and improve posture. The focus is on performing the moves and breathing in a slow, controlled fashion, which makes it a good way to unwind at the end of a long day. Many health clubs, gyms, and YMCAs offer tai chi classes, and this noncompetitive slower-paced class can help you decompress at the end of a hectic day.

ACTION

Sign up for an exercise class of your choosing and do it in place of one of your usual walks.

FEELING GOOD
the power of the pen

You've been keeping a *Food and Exercise Journal* for seven weeks now, writing down what you eat, and when, and keeping track of your workouts. Simply taking that step can help you meet your nutritional and fitness goals.

Taking your journal a step further and writing about your life, your feelings, your dreams, and your challenges offers additional benefits. This kind of more in-depth journaling can make a difference in the way you feel, help reduce anxiety and overcome grief, give you answers to problems, and provide you with insights into your life you may not have had before.

In fact, researchers are now finding that there are also health benefits to journaling. Keeping a journal has been shown to improve physical health, psychological well-being, and physiological functioning. It may be that writing down ways to deal with problems or expressing your feelings on the page reduces the amount of stress you feel. On a practical level, journaling can help you set goals and take time to reflect upon your life.

getting started

You don't need a fancy ink pen or an elegant diary to keep your journal—a simple notebook is all that's necessary. If you prefer something more upscale, bookstores offer dozens of different journals in all sizes, shapes, and covers. Some have lined paper; some have blank paper. Remember that what's important isn't the journal itself but what you do with it.

Make a note of the date and begin writing. You may want to start with what's happening in your life right now, or simply record the events of the day. You can use a journal to:

- Get in touch with your emotions and feelings.
- Track the events of your day-to-day life.
- Express thankfulness for all the good things you have in your life (some people keep "gratitude journals," where they list what they're thankful for).
- Determine your priorities and goals and track your progress toward them.
- Record your children's progress as they learn and grow.
- Get out frustrations and figure out ways to cope during stressful times.

There's no "right" or "wrong" when it comes to journaling. You can start a journal at any time of the year, or in connection with a particular event—the first of the year, the day you find out you're pregnant, or after you set a significant goal for yourself. Some people start a journal on January 1 and keep it every day; others write when they feel like it. Whatever you choose is up to you—that's all that matters.

what do i write about?

When you write is up to you. *What* you write is also your choice. You may want to use your journal as a place to express your frustrations with your job—better there than blowing up at your boss! Maybe you're considering making a big decision—

whether to move, or marry, or start your own business—and writing about it can help you see the pros and cons of all possible outcomes. Or maybe you simply want to write about what's happening in your life and use it as a chance to reflect.

Want to write, but you're stuck? Give these writing prompts a try:

- Write down five words that describe how you're feeling. Are you worried? Tired? Distracted? Comfortable? Content? Take one of those words and explore it. What are you worried about, for example? Why do you feel content?
- List five things in your life you're grateful for. They can be big or small— hearing your child's laugh in the morning, thick fluffy socks, or being healthy and strong.
- Describe your setting. Where are you? What does it look like? What does the room or place feel like? What do you like about it? What don't you like?
- Write down what you're not feeling, or doing, or seeing. Focusing on what's not there helps you see what is.
- Write down your goals. Make a list of what you'd like to accomplish in your life. Would you like to learn how to scuba dive? Take a ride in a hot-air balloon? Meet the president? Write a book? Swim with dolphins? Drive in a NASCAR race? Use your journal to dream. You may be surprised at what comes out.
- Instead of listing your goals, write down the achievements you're most proud of. What makes the list, and why? How has this impacted your life?
- Think about the people in your life. Write about how they've made a difference in yours. What effect are you having on their lives? Is it what you intend?
- Make a list of your favorites—favorite food, favorite movie, favorite book. What do they have in common? How often do you indulge in your favorites?
- Start with "I remember . . ." and write a memory. It can be anything—an event from your childhood, or something that happened last week.

You may decide to write every night, or you may only journal when you feel the need. Keeping your journal in a conspicuous place—on your nightstand, for example—will remind you to write in it, but you may also want to stash it in a secret place so no one else can read it. Keep it in a locked box, hide it, or ask the people around you not to read it. Even then, you may feel more comfortable using code words or secret names for some events or people in your life. You shouldn't have to worry about hurting someone's feelings in your journal—it should be a place that is just for you.

ACTION

You've already been keeping a *Food and Exercise Journal* to record your food intake and exercise program. In addition, as an option, write about anything you're feeling for 5 minutes a day. If you like, you can designate a separate notebook or diary as a journal and begin keeping it regularly.

action summary

EATING WELL
- Shop to replenish your healthy pantry.
- Eat regular meals and snacks, stopping when you are at a 5 or 6 on the hunger scale.
- Drink enough to stay well hydrated, including at least five glasses of water and a maximum of one sugary drink a day.
- Use healthy fats for cooking, dressings, and spreads.
- Eat two to four servings of fruit and three to six servings of vegetables each day.
- Check the ingredient list on your food labels.
- Get at least three servings of whole grains a day and limit refined grains.
- Record in your journal everything you eat and drink.

GETTING FIT
- Walk for 20 to 30 minutes 3 times at mid-intensity.
- Stretch and do strength training 3 times.
- Include a fun element in your fitness program.
- Sign up for a class.
- Note your activity in your journal.

FEELING GOOD
- Do the 5-minute breather or mini-vacation once a day.
- Practice mindfulness.
- Say "no" to tasks you don't want to and don't have to do.
- Keep up your bedtime ritual.
- Do a deep-relaxation or meditation exercise once.
- Optional:
  Tackle a clutter-clearing project.
  Explore journaling.

WEIGHT _____

THIS WEEK'S CHANGES:

1. Eat fish at least twice.

2. Try some more challenging strength-training moves.

3. Plan some special time with your partner or family (optional).

WEEK **9**

EATING WELL
go fish

Fish is one of those foods you either love or fear. If you already love fish, this week you will be happy to learn about its benefits and some new, healthy ways to prepare it. I'll also tell you which seafood is safest, and which you are better off avoiding. If you fear fish, whether it is because you are afraid it tastes "fishy" or because you haven't a clue how to buy it or cook it, this is the week to jump in and explore some seafood.

seafood: the good . . .

Seafood gives you lots of nutrition without a lot of calories, making it an ideal food if you're trying to stay trim (and who isn't, really?). It is an excellent source of high-quality protein, and it's rich in B vitamins and minerals like zinc, magnesium, and iron. Shellfish and fish like sole, cod, and catfish are extra lean and very low calorie. Fish such as salmon, sardines, and herring are higher in fat, but their fat content actually makes them an even bigger boon to your health.

The fat in fish—omega-3—gives it life-saving properties. This fat protects health by preventing blood clots, improving elasticity of blood vessels, lowering triglycerides and blood pressure, and boosting immunity. It also helps stabilize the rhythm of the heart. You can get omega-3 fat from other foods, as I mentioned in Week 5 (see page 97), but the most important types of omega-3 fat are only found in fish.

Study after study has shown that people who eat fish are less likely to suffer from heart disease and cancer. In one recent study women who ate two to four servings of fish a week were 31 percent less likely to develop heart disease than those who ate fish less than once a month. And in another study people who ate two or more servings of fish a week had a 30 to 50 percent less risk of certain cancers. There is also evidence that eating fish at least twice a week could ease the symptoms of rheumatoid arthritis.

. . . and the bad

That's the good news. Now here is the bad news: as our waters have become polluted with industrial waste like mercury, dioxins, and polychlorinated biphenyls

(PCBs), so have many of our fish. Mercury is of particular concern, since certain species of fish contain so much of the heavy metal they may actually be toxic. Scientists aren't sure how toxic the form of mercury in fish is to humans, but until more is known, it is best to play it safe.

Fish that live in waters contaminated with methylmercury, from power plants and other pollution sources, absorb mercury through their gills and get it from their food. The higher the fish is on the food chain, and the bigger it is, the more mercury it accumulates. So large fish like shark and swordfish harbor the most of this poisonous heavy metal.

When people consume excess mercury, it accumulates in the body and can harm the brain and nervous system. Children are especially vulnerable to mercury overload, as are fetuses, since their nervous systems are just developing. So, while eating fish can be a boon to your health, it is critical to choose the right kinds. That means eating seafood with low mercury levels and avoiding or limiting those with high mercury levels, especially if you are pregnant or nursing. (See the box below.) If you like to fish or have a fisherman in the family, you know there is nothing quite like freshly caught fish. But before you indulge, be sure to contact your state health department about the safety of the fish in your area.

the best and worst of the sea

USUALLY (eat two or more times a week) This seafood contains the lowest level of mercury:

	MERCURY	OMEGA-3
Anchovies*	low	highest
Catfish	low	low
Clams	low	low
Crab	low	low
Flounder/Sole	low	moderate
Herring*	low	highest
Lobster (spiny)	low	low
Oysters	low	high
Salmon*	low	highest
Sardines*	low	highest

*Women of childbearing age should limit these fish to two times a month, and opt for wild or canned salmon instead of farmed, whenever possible, to minimize exposure to PCBs and other contaminants.

USUALLY (CONTINUED)

Scallops	low	low
Shrimp	low	low
Squid	low	low
Tilapia	low	low
Trout (freshwater)	low	high
Whitefish	low	high

SOMETIMES (eat no more than once a week) This seafood has moderate levels of mercury:

	MERCURY	OMEGA-3
Bluefish	moderate	high
Cod	moderate	low
Halibut	moderate	low
Lobster (American)	moderate	low
Mahimahi	moderate	low
Perch (freshwater)	moderate	low
Sablefish	moderate	highest
Snapper	moderate	low
Tuna (canned light)	moderate	low

RARELY (eat no more than once a month) This seafood contains high mercury levels. Avoid if you are pregnant, nursing, or planning a pregnancy:

	MERCURY	OMEGA-3
Grouper	high	low
Orange roughy	high	low
Tuna (fresh, canned albacore)	high	low

AVOID (do not eat) This seafood has the highest mercury levels:

	MERCURY	OMEGA-3
King mackerel	highest	highest
Shark	highest	high
Swordfish	highest	moderate
Tilefish	highest	moderate

shellfish and cholesterol

Happily, most shellfish are low in mercury, but many people shun shellfish because they have heard they are high in cholesterol. It's true that some shellfish, especially squid and shrimp, are high in cholesterol. Three ounces of shrimp has 170 milligrams of cholesterol, a little more than half the 300-milligrams-per-day limit recommended by the American Heart Association; squid and crab are also relatively high in cholesterol. But the latest research shows that the cholesterol you eat isn't the main dietary factor influencing your blood cholesterol. Saturated fat is. Since shellfish has virtually no saturated fat (unless you dip it in butter!), it can easily be a part of heart-healthy eating. So feel free to enjoy it!

to market, to market

You belly up to the fish counter and stand there perplexed. You are thinking, Is this a good place to buy my fish? How do I know if it is fresh? Should I buy it frozen? How do I cook it once I get home? Will my kids like it? Maybe I should just get some hamburger. Before you give up, let me help.

First of all, step back and evaluate the vendor. The area should look and smell clean. Fish should be displayed on a thick bed of fresh, not melting, ice, and the seafood should be arranged with the bellies down so the melting ice drains away from the fish, reducing the chance of spoilage. The person behind the counter should be knowledgeable about different types of seafood and freely tell you how old the food is and explain why it is fresh.

The fish itself should have firm and shiny flesh that springs back when pressed. Whole fish should have bright red gills, clear eyes (some fish, like walleye, have naturally cloudy eyes, however), and be slime-free. The fish should smell like the sea, not fishy or ammonialike.

Frozen fish is also a good option, and an easy way to have seafood at your fingertips. I actually prefer to buy shrimp frozen, because they are usually shipped frozen and defrosted prior to sale at a fish counter anyway. They don't take long to defrost, so it is easy to boil some up on the spur of the moment, or toss a few into a jarred pasta sauce after you heat it (I like to add some spinach, too) for an effortless pasta dinner. Frozen fillets are also a good choice. They taste very fresh, as they are usually flash-frozen soon after being caught. Just be sure to buy plain fillets, not the breaded, fried kind.

Once you choose your fish, you will be surprised how quick and easy it is to prepare deliciously. The simplest thing to do is brush a fish fillet with a little olive oil, squeeze some lemon on it, add a little salt and pepper, and some tarragon, oregano, or other herb, if you'd like. Then just stick it under the broiler for 8 minutes per every inch of thickness. Grilling fish is also a cinch, but remember that flaky fish such as sole falls apart on the grill, so stick with salmon or shrimp for cooking out.

recipes

Each of the following fish dishes are quick and easy enough for beginners, yet special enough to impress guests.

citrus-ginger flounder with snow peas SERVES 4

4 small flounder fillets, 4 to 6 ounces each

4 cups snow peas (about ³/₄ pound)

¹/₂ cup Citrus-Ginger Dressing (page 102)

Lemon wedges

Preheat the oven to 425°F. Place each fish fillet on a large square of foil and turn up the edges of the foil. Top each fillet with 1 cup of snow peas and 2 tablespoons of dressing. Fold the foil around the fish to form a pouch and crimp it so it is sealed.

Put the foil pouches on a baking sheet and bake for 15–20 minutes, until fish flakes easily with a fork. Put the contents of each pouch on a plate and garnish with lemon. (This is great served over a bed of rice.)

Calories 214; Fat 6.4 g (Sat .7 g, Mono 3 g, Poly 1.9 g); Protein 28.6 g; Carb 9.5 g; Fiber 1.7 g; Chol 68 mg; Sodium 118 mg

poached salmon with mustard-dill sauce SERVES 4

4 salmon fillets, 4 to 6 ounces each

Mustard-Dill Sauce (page 102)

Pour 3 cups of water into a deep, nonstick skillet and bring to a boil. Add the salmon and more water if necessary to cover the fish completely. Cover the skillet and cook over a medium-low heat for about 10 minutes per inch of thickness of the fish. Transfer the salmon to a plate using 2 spatulas. Cover and chill in the refrigerator for 2 hours or more.

Spoon the sauce over the chilled salmon and serve.

Calories 280; Fat 15.4 g (Sat 3.1 g, Mono 5.5 g, Poly 5.6 g); Protein 30 g; Carb 2.6 g; Fiber 0 g; Chol 84.2 mg; Sodium 165 mg

cod with almond-shallot topping   SERVES 4

2 tablespoons olive oil

4 cod fillets, 4 to 6 ounces each

1 cup chopped shallot

1/2 cup almonds, chopped

1/3 cup finely chopped fresh flat-leaf parsley

2 tablespoons fresh lemon juice

Salt and freshly ground black pepper to taste

Heat 1 tablespoon of the oil in a large nonstick skillet on a medium flame. Place the fish in the pan and cook for about 8 minutes, or until the fish is cooked through, turning once. Transfer the fish to a plate and cover to keep warm.

Add the other tablespoon of oil and the shallot to the skillet and cook over moderate heat, stirring occasionally, for 3 to 4 minutes. Add the almonds and, stirring frequently, cook for 3 minutes more. Add the parsley, lemon juice, and salt and pepper to taste. Cook for 1 minute more. Spoon the topping over the fish and serve.

Calories 300; Fat 15.9 g (Sat 1.7 g, Mono 10.3 g, Poly 2.9 g); Protein 29.7 g; Carb 10.6 g; Fiber 1.9 g; Chol 61 mg; Sodium 81 mg

ACTION

Eat fish at least two times this week, choosing from the "Usually" or "Sometimes" list (pages 233–235).

advanced strength training

This week you'll learn some new strength-building exercises you can add to your repertoire. I'll also describe some fun, easy ways to keep challenging your body with strength training.

pump it up

In Week 6, I showed you how to make your walks more challenging by increasing their intensity. You can do the same thing with strength training.

Think of it this way. Say you do 1 set of 10 pushups 3 times a week. The first couple of weeks, it feels difficult. Then, as your muscles get stronger and used to the demands being placed on them, it begins to get easier. That's good, and it means that you're growing stronger. But as the exercise becomes easier, it also means that your body isn't being challenged as much anymore. Eventually you'll hit a plateau and stop seeing results.

You started with 1 set of 8 to 12 reps of the strength-building moves. By this time, that's probably gotten pretty easy. To challenge yourself, you can add a set or 2 (so you're doing 2 or 3 sets of the basic moves), change the order in which you do them, or try different exercises. This week, I've included a series of new moves that work your legs first, and then target your upper body. Start with 1 set of the moves and work up to 2 or 3. Or you can try this workout one day a week and your original strength-training workout the other two days, or any combination you like. The key is to keep your muscles guessing.

advanced strengthening moves

Lying hip raises (works muscles in the backs of the legs)
Lying on your back, raise up on your elbows; your head and chest will be off the ground. Keeping your right leg extended, bend your left leg and place your left foot flat on the ground. Pushing down with your left heel and elbows, lift your butt up, squeezing your glutes and hamstrings, and slowly return to your original position. Do 8 to 12 reps before switching to the other leg.

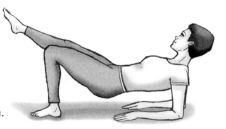

Two-position pushup (works chest muscles and backs of upper arms)

Assume a modified pushup position (lying flat, facing down, knees bent, weight on hands and knees) with both hands about 6 inches apart at breastbone level. Perform a pushup. When you return to the "up" position, move both hands (one at a time) so that they are slightly wider than shoulder-width apart, and perform a pushup from this wide position. (If you're strong enough, you can do this move in a standard pushup position, keeping your weight on your hands and toes instead of hands and knees.) Then move back to the original position and repeat. Do 8 to 12 reps.

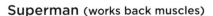

Superman (works back muscles)

Lie facedown with your arms straight out over your head. While pointing your toes and reaching out as far as you can with your arms and legs, slowly raise both arms and legs off the floor. (Don't lift your head or look up.) Hold for 3 breaths and release slowly. Perform 8 to 12 reps.

Supine single-arm extension
(works muscles on the back of your arms)

Lying faceup, hold a single dumbbell in your right hand and point your right arm straight up. Place 2 fingers of your left hand just below your right elbow, lightly touching your right triceps to help promote proper form. Keeping the upper arm still, slowly bend your right arm, letting the weight come down to your right shoulder before pressing it back up. Take 3 seconds to lower and 3 seconds to raise the weight; perform 8 to 12 reps.

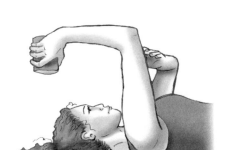

Sun gods (works shoulder muscles)

Stand up and place your arms out to your sides at shoulder height, palms facing down. Keeping your arms straight and your fingers pointed out, make 50 small, quick circles toward the front of your body; then make 50 circles toward the rear of your body. Move your arms to shoulder height in front of your body, palms facing down, and make 50 of the same tight circles to the inside, then 50 to the outside. Finally, raise your arms above your head, palms facing in, and make 50 tight circles in one direction and 50 in the other.

Controlled curls (works muscles in the front of your arms)

Hold a dumbbell or can in each hand. Standing straight with arms at your sides, slowly bring your arms up halfway to your shoulders (your lower arms will be parallel to the ground) in a half-curl, counting up for 4 seconds and down for 4 seconds; do 7 reps. Then do 7 reps from the halfway point to your shoulders, again using a 4-count. Finally, do 7 full curls using the 4-count up and down. (This move breaks a normal curl up into 2 distinct sections to work your biceps, the muscles in the front of your arms, differently.)

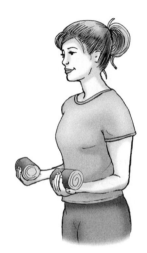

Laces (works stomach muscles)

Lie on your back with your knees bent and feet flat on the floor, arms at your sides. Lift both shoulders off the floor with your chin up and, with your left hand, reach toward the front of your left foot (where your shoelaces would be); then return to your original position and reach toward your "laces" on your right foot with your right hand. Alternate for 25 reps on each side.

circuit training

Circuit training has become increasingly popular. It combines cardiovascular activity with strength training, which makes it an effective way to burn calories and tone up at the same time—plus it's impossible to get bored because you're constantly switching activities. Yet you can significantly improve your cardiovascular fitness level by exercising in short bursts of approximately 60 seconds each.

Circuit training involves doing a "circuit" or series of strength-training exercises. Between each exercise, you jog, bike, jump rope, or otherwise stay active to keep your heart rate up, or you move immediately to the next exercise without resting. A circuit could be as simple as warming up, doing pushups, jogging in place for a

other ways to pump it up

Doing different exercises isn't the only way to give your body a new challenge. You can try these techniques as well:

MAKE IT LARGE Want to target your muscles in a short amount of time? Give what weight lifters call giant sets a try. With a giant set, you do two or three exercises in a row that use the same muscles—like doing lunges and then immediately doing squats afterward. It's more difficult because you're increasing the amount of work your muscles have to perform.

SLOW IT DOWN Recently, "super slow" strength training has come into favor. It's always good to do strength-training moves in a slow, controlled fashion—it eliminates momentum and forces your muscles to work harder. Try slowing down your reps even more—take 10 seconds to lift, and 10 seconds to return, for example. It's much more demanding.

WORK TO YOUR MAX Once your body gets stronger, you'll need to add more weights or more repetitions of an exercise to continue to challenge yourself. At the end of a set, your muscles should feel fatigued—if you feel like you could do another 5 or 10 reps, you're not working hard enough.

HIT THE CIRCUIT When you circuit train, you keep your heart rate high while doing different strength-training moves. It's a great way to add a cardiovascular component to your strength training.

minute, doing lunges, jogging in place for another minute, doing squats, jogging in place for a minute, doing crunches, warming down, and then repeating the whole sequence once or twice.

The difficulty (and effectiveness) of a session depends on many exercises you do, the speed and intensity at which you exercise, the length of intervals, the time you spend doing each exercise, and how many circuits you do. Basically, the greater the variety of activities, the better it is for overall fitness. Research shows that doing circuit training just once or twice a week can make a big difference in your fitness level. Give it a try to boost your regular routine.

Circuit training should be challenging but not exhausting. Work at a comfortable pace for you—your goal is to keep your heart rate up during the cardio portions of the circuit, but you don't want to collapse after 5 minutes. You may find it easier to push yourself, though, because you know you're going to switch to a different activity after only a minute. It's a flexible way to train—if time is limited, circuit training can count as both cardio and strength training.

Before you circuit train, walk for 5 minutes to warm up. Have any equipment you'll need (weights, for example) handy. Decide in advance what order you'll perform the exercises in—for example, you can use the workout in this chapter or the original strength-training workout. Then, instead of resting in between exercises, jog or walk briskly in place to keep your heart rate up. At the end of the circuit, cool down and perform your stretching exercises.

ACTION

Try the advanced strength-training workout, or experiment with circuit training.

family ties

reconnecting with your family

The key to happiness for most people doesn't turn on fame, fortune, or even career success. While these things may play a part in overall satisfaction, it's relationships with the people we love that are likely to have the biggest influence on our day-to-day satisfaction. Most of us realize that maintaining close relationships with those we love—especially our family—requires time and effort. Yet when time is in short supply, it's often our relationships, not our jobs or errands or even paying the bills, that suffer. We may schedule everything else in our lives, but we fail to make time for the people who are most important to us.

Take a minute to consider your relationships with your family members. Are your connections as close and meaningful as you would like them to be? Would you like to have more time to spend with those you love? Can you remember the last time you had a heart-to-heart talk with your children or spouse?

Think about ways you can reconnect. For example, it might be as simple as e-mailing your sister who lives out of state once a week, or planning a weekly no-TV family night to play games with your kids. What you do needn't be expensive or extravagant—there's simply no substitute for time with your family, especially your children. That doesn't mean you need to spend hours every day pondering the deepest questions of the universe with your teenager. You can have quality time during a trip to the grocery store or on the way home from school.

Connecting with kids Chances are you ask your children the same question day after day: "How was school today?" Instead, ask something different: "What was the best thing that happened to you today?" "So, who's your favorite teacher right now? Why?" "What was the toughest thing you had to do today?" "If you could go anywhere, where would you go?"

Ask questions and really *listen*. Set aside your natural urge to teach and help and protect. Don't try to correct your child. Just listen and connect.

Connecting with your partner We often take our partners or spouses for granted, and most of our conversations with them revolve around basics—who will pick up the kids from the birthday party, when to replace the roof of the house, locating lost keys. You've already made a date with your child or children. Do the same with your partner. You don't have to make it an expensive evening out—the idea is that once a week, you'll spend time together doing something fun and enjoying each other's company.

Connecting with your extended family With your parents, siblings, and other relatives, decide that you'll make more of an effort. Take it beyond the standard "how are you" and ask what's happening in their lives. Ask your parents and siblings to share memories with you. What are their hopes for the future? How are they spending their time? What's most important to them? Use e-mail and phone calls to stay in touch with distant family—or create a listserv, or group e-mail list, for your entire family to keep up on what's happening. Encourage your children to have relationships with their grandparents and other relatives, and look for ways to plan times to be together. It doesn't have to be over the holidays—a summer vacation or long weekend can be the perfect time for a family reunion or get-together.

ACTION

Make a commitment to plan a special time with your partner or family. Do something fun—maybe something you haven't tried before, like going hiking or visiting the zoo or in-line skating in the park. Remember, this change is optional.

action summary

EATING WELL

- Shop to replenish your healthy pantry.
- Eat regular meals and snacks, stopping when you are at a 5 or 6 on the hunger scale.
- Drink enough to stay well hydrated, including at least five glasses of water and a maximum of one sugary drink a day.
- Use healthy fats for cooking, dressings, and spreads.
- Eat two to four servings of fruit and three to six servings of vegetables each day.
- Check the ingredient list on your food labels.
- Get at least three servings of whole grains a day and limit refined grains.
- Eat fish at least twice this week.
- Record in your journal everything you eat and drink.

GETTING FIT

- Walk for 20 minutes 3 times at mid-intensity.
- Stretch and do strength training and core training 3 times.
- Include a fun element in your fitness program.
- Continue to attend a fitness class.
- Try advanced strengthening moves or circuit training.
- Note your activity in your journal.

FEELING GOOD

- Do the 5-minute breather or mini-vacation once a day.
- Practice mindfulness.
- Say "no" to tasks you don't want to and don't have to do.
- Keep up your bedtime ritual.
- Do a deep relaxation or meditation exercise at least once.
- Optional:
  Tackle a clutter-clearing project.
  Explore journaling.
  Plan a special time with your partner or family.

WEIGHT _____

THIS WEEK'S CHANGES:

1. **Eat a serving of nuts, seeds, beans, or soy each day.**

2. **Increase the intensity of your walking.**

3. **Reconnect with a friend** (optional).

WEEK

10

a new food group: nuts, seeds, and legumes

There's nothing like the fun of shelling and eating peanuts at a ball game, ladling up some hearty bean chili on a cold winter's day, or sprinkling on your favorite nuts to spice up an otherwise dull salad. Think these can be only occasional indulgences? Nope—they're treats you don't have to feel guilty about. Nuts, seeds, and legumes (beans, lentils, dried peas, peanuts, and soy) are incredibly healthy and can help you keep your weight in check. This week we're going to get a little nutty (and "bean-y") as we explore ways to get more of these delicious nuggets into your life.

Because they are great sources of protein, nuts, seeds, and legumes have traditionally been lumped as a "meat alternative" into the same basic food group as meat. But emerging science reveals that these protein-packed plants offer so many unique health benefits that they should be much more than meat's understudy—in fact, they should be on the main stage. These vegetable proteins are so important, I believe they deserve a food group of their very own, so I have given them one in the *Small Changes, Big Results* eating plan.

I am not the first to grant nuts, seeds, and legumes their own food group. The folks at the National Institutes for Health did it when they created their DASH (Dietary Approaches to Stop Hypertension) Diet. Studies proved that this eating plan dramatically reduced blood pressure in only two weeks! The DASH diet is similar to the one I'm discussing here: a plan that is rich in fruits, vegetables, whole grains, low-fat dairy products, lean meats, poultry, fish, and the headliner of this week's chapter, a new sixth food group: nuts, seeds, and legumes.

There are reams of evidence supporting the health benefits of these wonderful foods. As a whole, they are all great sources of protein, fiber, potassium, zinc, and magnesium. Individually, they each have different properties that protect your health and expand your mealtime options.

go a little nuts (and seeds)

Nuts used to be considered a sinful treat, high in fat and calories—a food nibbled guiltily in a bar or at holiday parties. Well, you can erase any notion of nuts as a no-no, because nuts (including tree nuts like almonds, walnuts, and hazelnuts as well as peanuts, which are a nutlike legume), nut butters, and seeds are just plain good for you.

Check this out: nuts are loaded with healthy monounsaturated fat, which has been shown to lower bad cholesterol and help keep blood sugar steady. (Flax seeds and walnuts also contain hard-to-get omega-3 fats.) Nuts are chock-full of important nutrients like vitamin E, magnesium, calcium, zinc, copper, iron, and of course protein. Plus they are packed with protective phytochemicals and fiber. There is so much evidence that eating nuts reduces the risk of heart disease that the Food and Drug Administration even lets nut packagers boast about it on their labels.

Because they are such a satisfying food, nuts and seeds can also help you manage your weight. A small handful of nuts and a piece of fruit can help you get past those afternoon sweets cravings and give you the stamina you need to get in some exercise or make it through the rest of your day. They're also an ideal on-the-go snack you can stash in your bag or desk drawer until hunger calls.

One thing, though: notice I said a *small* handful. Nuts, nut butters, and seeds are high in calories, so if you suddenly start eating piles of nuts or scoops of peanut butter out of the jar in addition to what you are already consuming, you will probably gain weight. The trick is to substitute a small portion of nuts—say, about $1/3$ cup nuts, $1/4$ cup seeds, or 2 tablespoons of nut butter—*instead* of less healthy options. So grab a handful of almonds and a piece of fruit instead of a candy bar or chips in the afternoon. Spread some peanut butter on your toast in the morning in lieu of butter or cream cheese. Or toss some pumpkin seeds on your salad at lunch instead of bacon bits or cheese, both of which are high in saturated fat.

cool beans

The variety of dishes that start with the simple little bean is astounding. Nearly every culture around the world boasts a delicious and unique bean dish. Think about it—there are red beans and rice in South America; dahl, an Indian lentil stew; Middle Eastern hummus (pureed chickpeas); black-eyed peas and rice in the West Indies; Italian *pasta e fagioli* (pasta and white beans); and edamame (young soy beans) in

Japan. Some North American favorites include baked beans, hopping john (black-eyed peas), and traditional bean chili. Then there are the soups—lentil, split pea, white bean and garlic, navy bean, minestrone. The list goes on. If you think eating healthfully has to be boring or you yawn just thinking about another plain chicken breast, wake up to any of these exciting bean dishes.

People have gotten so creative with beans and other legumes like dried peas and lentils because they have all been a dietary staple for centuries. They're inexpensive and easy to prepare, yet provide essential protein, B vitamins, zinc, copper, magnesium, iron, potassium, fiber, and antioxidants. They are also one of the best sources of folate, the B vitamin we now know prevents birth defects and guards against heart disease. One cup of beans provides almost a full day's worth of folate! Plus beans have virtually no fat, and they are incredibly satisfying, which means you can feel comfortably full eating beans without packing on the calories.

Beans are sometimes shunned as a poor man's food, providing cheap protein for those who can't afford meat. But thanks to the bean's incredible nutrient profile, people who get more of their protein from beans, and less from fatty meats, will find they are much richer health-wise.

So next time you crave Mexican food, skip the beef tacos and go for the bean burrito instead. Try a filling, fragrant bowl of split pea or lentil soup for lunch, or sprinkle some garbanzo beans, also known as chickpeas, on your salad. Premade hummus—pureed chickpeas with garlic and sesame paste—is a staple in my fridge. It makes for an excellent lunch on the run. Just spread some on a whole wheat pita, stuff in some prewashed greens, and you've got a portable, filling sandwich.

While it's easy to prepare dried beans, they do take time. Dried beans need to be soaked overnight and then cooked for 1 to 4 hours. I usually don't think that far ahead, so I keep a variety of canned beans at my fingertips. Yes, canned beans are fairly high in salt, whereas dried beans have almost none. But rinsing canned beans under cold water gets rid of almost half the sodium, and you can't beat the convenience. Some quick meal ideas: toss a can of white beans into your pasta sauce while it is heating; sauté chopped onion, garlic, and green peppers, add a can of black beans, and serve over rice (see recipe on page 33); or substitute half the meat in your favorite beef chili recipe with red beans (use one 16-ounce can of beans per pound of meat).

Okay, I know you're thinking it, so let's be frank. You say you avoid beans because they give you gas? Well, there are ways to minimize this uncomfortable side effect (or should I say sound effect?). First, if you haven't had beans in a while, don't dig into a big bean-y bowl of chili just yet. Start with a small bowl. You want to introduce beans into your diet gradually, so your body has a chance to adapt.

If you use dried beans, draining and rinsing them after soaking eliminates some of the gas-causing compounds. Cooking your beans thoroughly also helps. Canned beans are usually already well cooked; rinsing them before you prepare them eliminates a lot of the "gas factor." Once you have built up your tolerance, enjoy beans regularly. You're less likely to suffer from gas when your body is used to these fiber-rich foods. Another option is to try Beano, an over-the-counter supplement that helps reduce gas. It contains enzymes that reduce the amount of gas your body produces and the accompanying discomfort along with it. You simply shake a few drops onto your first bite of beans or other gas-producing foods.

beyond tofu

Soybeans are legumes like those I've been talking about. But soy has such unique properties that it is often considered a class all its own. In the past years, soy has become increasingly popular and there are now dozens of soy-based foods including tofu, soy milk, tempeh (a savory soybean cake), soy nuts, soy cheese, and miso (a rich soybean paste used for flavoring). Now you can even buy soy burgers, soy hot dogs, soy "chicken" nuggets, and, believe it or not, soy bacon.

Soy has been making big headlines recently. First it was being hyped as a miracle food, and then it was decried as potentially dangerous. What's the bottom line? First, soy has numerous benefits. It has been shown to reduce cholesterol, fight certain cancers, and help prevent osteoporosis; it also may alleviate the symptoms of menopause in some women. And according to the FDA, 25 grams of soy protein a day (about four servings' worth of tofu or soybeans) has been shown to reduce the risk of heart disease.

But soy is not a miracle cure. In fact, when eaten in excess, soy can have some negative effects for people with a history of breast cancer, thyroid problems, or kidney stones. So while a daily serving or two of soy is a healthy addition to just about anyone's diet, it's a good idea to check with your doctor before loading up on more than that.

Soy is chock-full of nutrients like B vitamins, minerals, fiber, and healthy fats. But soy's benefits are mainly attributed to the type of protein it contains along with a powerful group of compounds called isoflavones. Different soy foods have varying amounts of naturally occurring protein and isoflavones. Soy flour, soy nuts, soybeans, soy milk, tempeh, and tofu are among the best sources. More processed foods, like that soy bacon I mentioned, generally have less but are still good sources.

Many food manufacturers have isolated soy protein and isoflavones and supplement their foods with one or both to try to give them soy's health edge. Nowadays you can buy soy-supplemented cereals, energy bars, and smoothie mix. But soy protein and isoflavones do the most good when they occur naturally, as opposed to when they are added. And it is easier to go overboard with supplements.

While there's no question that soy is good for you, cooking—and eating—soy can be intimidating. Many people assume they won't like it or don't know how to cook it. There are plenty of user-friendly, tasty soy foods out there. Simply grill up a delicious soy burger just as you would grill a beef burger. You can even get your soy without having to cook at all. Soy milk is delicious in a shake or on cereal. Soy nuts are a crunchy and flavorful snack on their own and make a great salad topping as well.

for vegetarians (and those who love them)

If you are a vegetarian (or someone you love is), you'll want to pay special attention to the foods highlighted this week—nuts, seeds, beans, and soy. They are often the protein mainstays of the vegetarian's diet.

While animal sources of protein contain all of the essential amino acids our bodies need, no single plant source can provide all the essential amino acids in quantities we need. However, certain foods "complement" one another to offer complete protein—in other words, eating both types of foods provides your body with all of the essential amino acids it needs. Nuts, seeds, beans, and soy are rich in the amino acids (protein's building blocks) that grains lack, and vice versa. Most vegetarians I know get plenty of grains but fall woefully short in the nut, seed, and bean category. It is critical to have both complementary groups in your diet each day, although you don't need to consume them at the same meal, as was once thought.

Are you thinking that if you eat cheese and milk, you needn't worry about consuming beans? Wrong. While milk products offer a complete protein and provide lots of calcium and vitamin D, they are poor sources of zinc and iron, minerals that many vegetarians fall short of. Nuts, seeds, beans, and soy are excellent sources of these essential minerals. So whether you are a vegan (someone who eats no animal products) or a lacto-ovo vegetarian (someone who eats no meat, fish, or poultry but consumes eggs and dairy products), you need to get at least two or three servings from the nuts, seeds, beans, and soy group every day.

That big, white, tasteless block of tofu may make the average home cook run away in fear. But tofu takes on the flavors of its marinade beautifully and is remarkably easy to prepare. (See Marinated Tofu, page 186.) And to make life even easier, many stores now carry premarinated, precooked tofu that you can simply cut up for salads, stir-fries, casseroles, or whatever.

Finally, don't forget one of my favorite soy foods, edamame, which are young natural soybeans, found either in the pod or shelled. They are often sold frozen and are perfect to have on hand at home—to prepare them, you simply boil them for about 5 minutes. Served in the pod, they are a wonderful healthy finger food. You just work the beans out of the pod with your teeth, eat the beans, and discard the empty pod. You can use shelled edamame just as you would any other bean, in salads, stews, and soups. With all these easy options, there is no reason not to give soy a try.

recipes

lentil soup SERVES 8 TO 10

This hearty soup makes a satisfying main dish. Serve it with a green salad and some whole-grain bread.

2 tablespoons olive oil
1 large onion, diced
4 carrots, diced
2 celery stalks, diced
1 garlic clove, minced
1/4 teaspoon dried thyme
2 bay leaves
2 1/2 cups lentils

12 cups (2 48-ounce cans) low-sodium chicken broth or vegetable broth
2 cups chopped fresh spinach, chard, or kale
1 tablespoon balsamic vinegar
Salt and freshly ground black pepper to taste

In a large soup pot, heat the olive oil over a medium-high flame. Add the onion, carrots, and celery and cook until they begin to soften, about 3 minutes. Add the garlic and cook for 1 more minute. Stir in the thyme, bay leaf, and lentils. Add the broth and bring to a boil.

Simmer on low heat for 1 hour. Add the chopped greens and vinegar and simmer for another 30 minutes. Season with salt and pepper to taste and serve.

Calories 325; Fat 7.1 g (Sat 2 g, Mono 3 g, Poly 1 g); Protein 23.9 g; Carb 44.5 g; Fiber 20.8 g; Chol 7.5 mg; Sodium 246 mg

white chili SERVES 6

Chili is a great party food. Just keep a pot of it warm on the stove, put out the fixin's, and let everyone help themselves.

2 tablespoons olive oil
1 pound boneless chicken breast, cut into bite-sized chunks
1 large onion, diced
3 garlic cloves, minced
2 4-ounce cans of chopped mild green chilis, undrained
1/2 cup tomatillo salsa (also called salsa verde), mild, medium, or hot, to taste
1 14 1/2-ounce can of low-sodium chicken broth

1/4 teaspoon ground cumin
1/2 teaspoon dried oregano
2 16-ounce cans of white beans, like cannellini, drained and rinsed
3 tablespoons lime juice
1/2 cup fresh cilantro, chopped
1 cup nonfat plain yogurt
1/2 cup shredded reduced-fat cheddar cheese

Heat 1 tablespoon of the oil in a large saucepan over a medium-high flame. Add the chicken and sauté for 5 minutes, or until cooked through. Remove from the pan and set aside. Add the remaining tablespoon of oil and the onion to the pan and sauté over medium heat until the onion is tender, about 3 minutes. Add the garlic and sauté for 1 minute more. Add the chilis, salsa, chicken broth, cumin, and oregano and bring to a boil. Reduce the heat and simmer for 20 minutes. Add the chicken and beans and cook for 5 minutes more. Stir in the lime juice. Serve topped with cilantro, yogurt, and cheese.

Calories 317; Fat 8.1 g (Sat 1.6 g, Mono 3.8 g, Poly .7 g); Protein 33.2 g; Carb 37.8 g; Fiber 10.5 g; Chol 48 mg; Sodium 964 mg

marinated tofu SERVES 4

This baked tofu is crispy on the outside, creamy inside, and loaded with flavor. Removing as much water as possible from the tofu before cooking it, as in this recipe, helps the tofu absorb the flavors of the marinade and makes it cook up crisp rather than mushy. You can serve this hot or cold. It is delicious eaten as is, or in sandwiches, salads, or stir-fries. (See recipe on page 221.)

1 pound extra-firm tofu
2 tablespoons low-sodium soy sauce
1 tablespoon orange juice

2 teaspoons sesame oil
1 teaspoon canola oil
Cooking spray

Slice the tofu into $1/2$-inch-thick slabs and lay the slices on top of paper towels. Use more paper towels to firmly pat the tofu in order to remove as much of the water as possible. This should take about 3 paper towels and should take 2 minutes. Cut the tofu into cubes.

In a medium bowl, combine the soy sauce, orange juice, sesame oil, and canola oil. Add the tofu cubes and toss gently. Cover and let the tofu marinate in the refrigerator for at least 30 minutes, and up to 24 hours.

Preheat the oven to 450°F. Spray a large shallow baking dish with cooking spray. Place the tofu in a single layer in the baking dish. Bake for 25 to 30 minutes, or until golden brown.

Calories 145; Fat 10.4 g (Sat 1.4 g, Mono 3.1 g, Poly 5.3 g); Protein 12.3 g; Carb 3.4 g; Fiber .5 g; Chol 0 mg; Sodium 311 mg

mixed vegetables with peanut sauce SERVES 4

This is a rich, satisfying meal that gets its protein from peanuts. Serve over rice.

1 teaspoon canola oil

1 large garlic clove, minced

$1/2$ cup natural-style creamy peanut butter

$1/8$ teaspoon cayenne pepper

1 tablespoon cider vinegar or white-wine vinegar

1 tablespoon honey

2 tablespoons low-sodium soy sauce

$1/4$ teaspoon salt

3 cups string beans

4 large carrots, cut on the diagonal into thin rounds

1 large head broccoli, cut into spears

1 teaspoon toasted sesame oil

$1/2$ cup chopped scallions

Heat the canola oil in a medium saucepan over a medium flame. Reduce the heat to low, add the garlic, and sauté until fragrant, about 1 minute. Stir in the peanut butter, cayenne pepper, vinegar, honey, soy sauce, salt, and $1^{1}/2$ cups water, mixing thoroughly. The mixture will be clumpy at first but will become creamy as it heats up and with additional stirring. Simmer on the lowest possible heat for 30 minutes, stirring occasionally.

Meanwhile, steam the string beans, carrots, and broccoli in a large steamer for about 15 minutes, or until tender.

Arrange the cooked vegetables on a plate and top with the peanut sauce. Drizzle with sesame oil and garnish with scallions.

Calories 336; Fat 19.4 g (Sat 3.7 g, Mono 8.9 g, Poly 5.6 g); Protein 16 g; Carb 33.6 g; Fiber 12 g; Chol 0 mg; Sodium 669 mg

Include at least one serving of nuts, beans, seeds, or soy in your diet each day. One serving is ½ cup cooked beans or tofu, 1 cup soy milk, ⅓ cup nuts, ¼ cup seeds, or 2 tablespoons nut butter.

GETTING FIT
walking to the max

You've been walking regularly for more than two months now and have learned how to increase your intensity from low to medium. This week, you'll learn how to ratchet up to high intensity.

walking to the max

A few weeks ago, I explained how to take your cardiovascular exercise up a notch and make it more intense. You'll recall that you can do this by increasing the amount of time you exercise, the intensity at which you exercise, or the grade you're walking on (it's more difficult walking up a steep slope than a flat surface).

Most people are comfortable doing low- to moderate-intensity exercise; it's challenging but not too difficult. Once your body has become accustomed to moderate-intensity exercise, however, you can reap even more benefits by adding some high-intensity sessions to your workout program.

High-intensity exercise burns more calories per minute than low- or moderate-intensity exercise because you're placing more demands on your cardiovascular system and your muscles. Your body must work harder, so you burn more calories. High-intensity exercise also elevates your metabolism more than a moderate-intensity workout and has a greater "afterburn effect," meaning that your body burns even more calories after exercise than it would normally.

Competitive athletes and other highly trained exercisers may do high intensity two or three times a week; however, for most people, one or two high-intensity sessions a week is more than enough. Again, if you're exercising 3 times a week at moderate intensity, that's great. If you're ready to take it up a notch, choose one of these options:

- Walk for 40 minutes at mid-intensity; or
- Walk for 30 minutes, including some "intervals," or bursts, where you walk as fast as you can (that makes it high-intensity exercise); or
- Walk for 30 minutes with hills; or
- Walk and run for 30 minutes.

interval training

Doing intervals will not only make your workouts more challenging, you'll also burn additional calories and improve your overall fitness in the process. When you do intervals, you purposely increase your intensity for short bursts of time, interspersing those bursts with rest or recovery periods. By doing so, your body is forced to work much harder than it's used to, and that's the whole point.

While athletes use intervals to drop their times and win competitions, interval training pays benefits to even everyday exercisers. First, it forces you to use your fast-twitch muscle fibers, which may not be used during low- or moderate-intensity exercise. (Your muscles contain both "fast-twitch" and "slow-twitch" fibers, which are recruited depending on what type of activity you do. Long, slow, aerobic exercise usually depends on slow-twitch fibers, while more intense exercise relies on fast-twitch fibers.) Second, interval training helps make your heart stronger and improves your ability to use oxygen efficiently.

Interval training also burns calories at a faster rate than exercising at a slower pace. If you intersperse a few intervals throughout your normal cardio work, you'll burn more calories during the exercise itself as well as afterward due to the "afterburner" effect.

Ready to try some interval training of your own? You can do intervals during your regular cardio workout, whether it's walking, jogging, cycling, rowing, or climbing stairs. All you need is a watch to track the interval times.

As with any cardio workout, warm up first. You may also want to do some stretches after your warm-up, but before you begin the intervals. Remember that you're going to be working harder than normal and recruiting fast-twitch muscles, so you may feel out of breath and your muscles may "burn" a little.

A 1:1 ratio is usually a good place to begin. For example, you might walk slowly for 5 minutes to warm up, and then walk as fast as you can for 1 minute, then walk slowly for 1 minute, and repeat 5 times; then finish the workout at your usual pace to cool down. As you get fitter, you can extend the effort times—for example, by walking fast for 2 minutes, walking slow for 1 minute. Or you may want to do your usual workout for 20 minutes or so and then add intervals at the end (they can be tiring).

ready to run?

Many walkers are happy continuing to walk for fitness. They make their walks more challenging by increasing their speed or distance, or add hills or inclines to work harder. Others get bitten by the running bug and decide they'd like to try jogging or running instead.

Running is a more demanding physical activity than walking, but at this point, you should be ready for a new challenge. Start off by walking to warm up. After 5 or 10 minutes, begin to run slowly for a minute or so; then walk for a minute or until you catch your breath. Run again for a minute, then walk a minute. Maintain this routine for 30 minutes.

When you run, your head should be up, your chest lifted, arms relaxed at your sides. Don't let your head and shoulders hang forward as you tire; maintain proper posture as you run. You should be running heel to toe (that is, your heel strikes the ground first, then you roll onto your toes to push off) and your steps should be light. If you're slapping the ground, make an effort to run "lighter."

Depending on how you feel, you can increase your running sessions from 1:1 (running 1 minute, walking 1 minute) to 2:1 (running 2 minutes, walking 1 minute) and so on as you become fitter. Work up to 20 to 30 minutes of easy running over time.

ready, set, hike!

Hiking is another way to boost the intensity of your regular walks. Hiking or trail walking is usually more challenging than walking because you're covering rougher, often hilly terrain. The beauty of hiking, though, is that it gives you a chance to slow down and reconnect with nature while you move your body.

Hiking forces you to work harder because you're negotiating inclines and rougher footing than you may be used to. The faster you walk, the tougher it gets, but you can also choose to simply stroll. Either way, you'll be targeting the major muscles in your legs—your quadriceps, hamstrings, calves, and glutes.

Finding a place to hike is often easier than you might think. Local, state, and national parks are all good places. Some have maps and marked trails; some do not.

If you're new to hiking, stick to shorter, well-marked trails. With elevation changes, you may find a 2-mile hike more challenging than a 3-mile walk on a flat surface.

While you can usually wear the same clothes you walk in to hike in, bring along a jacket or other outer layer in case it gets chilly while you're hiking—the weather can change quickly, especially if you're hiking at higher altitudes. The same rules about layering clothes apply: start with a T-shirt or tank top if the weather's warm, but take along an extra layer or two. You may also want to wear hiking shoes or boots, which are designed to give better traction on slippery trails or rough terrain. Their thick soles will also protect your feet from rocks and other objects on the trail.

Depending on how long you'll hike, you'll also want to take along a backpack or fanny pack. Plan to take more food and more water than you think you'll need—it's better to be overprepared than underprepared. Bring water, easily portable food like trail mix, energy bars, or fruit, a plastic bag for garbage, a flashlight, a map, and a compass if you'll be walking on unmarked trails. A simple first-aid kit that contains an Ace bandage, Band-Aids, antiseptic spray, and a cell phone for emergencies is also a good idea.

Finally, check the weather forecast before you go. A little rain won't hurt you, but you don't want to be hiking in an electrical storm or other severe weather.

check out cross-training

Do any activity day in, day out, and you're bound to get bored. Cross-training—performing other types of exercise in addition to or instead of your usual one—helps prevent burnout, reduces your risk of injuries, and constantly challenges your body, which means more results from your program.

If you usually walk, you might cross-train with bicycling, swimming, or rowing—each activity uses different muscle groups in a different way. Even if you have a favorite cardio activity, do something different at least one day a week. You might use the bike instead of an elliptical trainer, or substitute a rowing workout for time on the stair machine.

Trying something new also makes you less likely to get bored—exercise isn't automatic, so you have to focus more on what you're doing. Because you're focusing on your workout rather than distracting yourself (or counting the minutes that are left), you're also more likely to get into a flow state, where you're thinking of nothing but what you're doing—which is a great mental release as well as a physical one.

ACTION

This week, do at least one of your three walks at high intensity by increasing the speed you walk at, the time you're walking, or adding more hills or inclines to your walk. If you like, you can choose to go hiking instead.

reconnecting with friends

Last week, I talked about the importance of maintaining close relationships with your family members. This week, I want you to think about the relationships you have with the other people in your life—your friends, coworkers, neighbors, and others you have daily contact with. Who do you consider your friends? Would you like closer relationships with them, or to spend more time with them?

Research shows that friendships not only enhance your life, but also protect and improve your health. And studies show that the happiest people are those who have both good mental health and good social relationships.

Some people have one or two close friends and a large circle of acquaintances; others have an extended group of people they're close to. Over time, new friendships are made through circumstance or shared interests while others are lost. It's natural to put our jobs and families ahead of our friends, but making time for people who you connect with and can laugh and share your life with only enriches your life.

Friendships take time and tending the same way that your relationships with your family do. Keeping in touch—whether by phone, e-mail, letters, or get-togethers—is an essential part of staying close. Make time for friends, and treat them with respect and consideration.

outgrowing a friend

It may be that the two of you used to be close and now feel that you don't have much in common anymore. Or perhaps things have happened that make you feel as though the friendship isn't worth your time. Think about your relationship with the person. Does she support you, believe in you, have your best interests in mind? Do you enjoy talking to her and spending time with her? Everyone has down days, but if you're sapped by speaking to her for even a few minutes, it may be time to end the relationship. (I call these people energy vampires because they're so good at draining you!) You can tell your friend that you just don't feel that you have much in common anymore, or simply stop calling or e-mailing. He or she will get the message. Remember, too, that ending a relationship that isn't good for you anymore makes more time in your life for people who will bring you joy and pleasure.

If this is a relationship that's really important to you, you may want to talk to your friend about the problem before you end it. Tell her how you feel and ask if there's a way to reconnect. Maybe there's something going on in her life that has affected her—something you don't know about. You won't know unless you ask.

ACTION

This week, if you like, make an effort to reconnect with someone you're close to but haven't spoken to in a while.

about forgiveness

The saying goes: to err is human, to forgive divine. Forgiving someone when he or she has hurt you can be extremely difficult. True forgiveness can set the stage for a deeper relationship, help prevent disagreements about inconsequential things, and improve your own health. Studies show that forgiveness is good for the heart as well as the soul. Harboring a grudge or resentment against someone or something can only have a negative effect on your health. Forgiving someone can release this negative energy and positively impact how you feel.

Many people find writing a letter to the person who hurt them is helpful. Get out all your feelings and frustrations on paper. Pretend you're in front of the person and this is your chance to tell them everything. Then rip the letter into tiny pieces or burn it. (Or, try talking to someone close to you about what happened to let you vent and gain perspective.)

Then make a conscious effort to let it go—after you've forgiven someone, don't keep bringing up the same incident. Dwelling on it, especially with the other person, may prevent you from really forgiving.

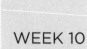

WEEK 10
action summary

EATING WELL
- Shop to replenish your healthy pantry.
- Eat regular meals and snacks, stopping when you are at a 5 or 6 on the hunger scale.
- Drink enough to stay well hydrated, including at least five glasses of water and a maximum of one sugary drink a day.
- Use healthy fats for cooking, dressings, and spreads.
- Eat two to four servings of fruit and three to six servings of vegetables each day.
- Check the ingredient list on your food labels.
- Get at least three servings of whole grains a day and limit refined grains.
- Eat fish at least twice this week.
- Eat at least one serving of nuts, seeds, beans, or soy each day.
- Record in your journal everything you eat and drink.

GETTING FIT
- Walk for 20 to 40 minutes 3 times at mid- or high intensity.
- Stretch and do strength training and core training 3 times.
- Include a fun element in your fitness program.
- Continue to attend a fitness class.
- Note your activity in your journal.

FEELING GOOD
- Do the 5-minute breather or mini-vacation once a day.
- Practice mindfulness.
- Say "no" to tasks you don't want to and don't have to do.
- Keep up your bedtime ritual.
- Do a deep relaxation or meditation exercise at least once.
- Optional:
  Tackle a clutter-clearing project.
  Continue journaling.
  Plan a special time with your partner or family.
  Reconnect with a friend.

WEIGHT _____

THIS WEEK'S CHANGES:

1. Switch to lean meats.

2. Increase the activity in your everyday life.

3. Do something to pamper your body (optional).

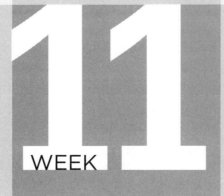

WEEK

EATING WELL
keep it lean

This week's "Eating Well" focus is one of the most convincing cases for the power of small changes. Amazingly, you can lose more than 6 pounds a year by making this one simple change: choosing a lean meat over a high-fat one each day.

For example, if you have 3 ounces of skinless chicken breast for dinner instead of the same amount of T-bone steak, you save about 60 calories. That might not sound like a lot, but over the course of a year that adds up to 21,900 calories, which translates into a 6-pound weight loss. The numbers are even more impressive when you consider that most people typically eat much more than 3 ounces of meat at dinner. After all, a restaurant-sized serving is about 10 ounces—or even more!

I know, I know: you probably already realize chicken breast is healthy and try to swap your red meat for white when you can. But if now you feel like you are going to start clucking if you eat much more chicken, take heart. Chicken is only one of many lean-meat options you can include on your "Usually" list. You may be surprised at the variety of meats—even red meats—and poultry that make the low-fat grade. Give them a try and they can make healthy eating less of a bore and add more variety to your diet.

protein power

Last week I talked about vegetarian sources of protein like nuts, seeds, beans, and legumes. When most people think of protein, though, they think of animal sources like beef, pork, and poultry, which, along with eggs, are our focus this week.

Protein is an essential part of your diet, and critical to the health of every cell in your body. It helps build, repair, and maintain body tissue like muscle and is used to create red blood cells as well as to keep your hair, skin, and fingernails healthy. It's responsible for helping produce antibodies that fight off bacteria, viruses, and germs and keeps your immune system running strong—studies show that people low on protein are more likely to get sick than people who eat enough of this nutrient. Also, low-fat protein foods are a boon to weight watchers because protein foods tend to be among the most satisfying, making you feel full on fewer calories.

Most Americans get plenty of protein, but new research points to the possibility that many people over age fifty may not be getting enough. The Recommended Dietary Allowance for protein is 50 grams for women and 63 grams for men, but many experts contend that 70 to 100 grams of protein a day may be beneficial for older people, especially when it comes to maintaining healthy bones.

Ideally you want to get your protein from both vegetable sources (like beans, soy, nuts, and grains) and animal sources (like meat, poultry, fish, eggs, and dairy). The key is making sure you get your animal protein without too much saturated fat.

high-protein foods

FOOD	PROTEIN (GRAMS)
Meat, poultry, and fish (3 ounces cooked)	20–30
Cottage cheese, low-fat (1/2 cup)	14
Yogurt, low-fat (1 cup)	12
Tofu, firm (1/2 cup)	10–20
Milk, low-fat (1 cup)	8
Peanut butter (2 tablespoons)	8
Beans, cooked (1/2 cup)	7
Egg, hard-boiled (1 egg)	6
Pasta, cooked (1/2 cup)	3
Bread (1 slice)	3

red doesn't always mean stop

One of the most nutrient-dense sources of protein is red meat, but it's often blamed for much of the heart disease and expanding waistlines in this country. It is true that most cuts of red meat, including beef, pork, and lamb, are laden with saturated fat and calories—major contributors to heart disease, obesity, and other problems. And as a whole, we eat far too much of it, from burgers and ribs to steaks and chops. Most people would be better off getting less protein from animal sources and more from vegetable sources and fish, as you have been doing in recent weeks. But to its credit, red meat is also full of key nutrients: zinc, iron, selenium, magnesium, and

B vitamins. When you choose the leanest cuts, meat is actually quite a dietary bargain, giving you a wealth of nutrition per calorie.

Choosing lean cuts of red meat is easier than you might think. The leanest cuts of pork and beef tend to have *loin* or *round* in their name, so read labels carefully. For example, beef top round, beef eye round, and pork tenderloin are the trimmest of the bunch, coming remarkably close to being as lean as skinless chicken breast. As you'll see in the chart on pages 200–202, other cuts of beef, pork, and some cuts of lamb are also reasonably low-fat choices.

The first step is to start with a lean cut of meat, but there are other things you can do to make your meal even slimmer. First, choose a "select" grade of meat, which has less fat marbled throughout the flesh than choice or prime grades. Then, trim off all visible fat, and use a cooking method that doesn't add extra fat to the dish—and in fact allows excess fat from the meat to drip off during cooking. Broiling, grilling, roasting on a rack, or stir-frying with just a little oil are good ways to reduce the fat content.

the "skinny" on ground beef

When buying ground beef, don't be fooled by labels boasting "85% lean." That label may sound good, but it is actually very high in fat. They are talking about percent lean by *weight,* not by calories. Meat that says *85% lean* actually gets about half its calories from fat. Only ground beef that is 90 to 95 percent lean qualifies as a "Usually" food.

You can eliminate about two thirds of the fat in ground beef with this drain-and-blot method: after browning the meat, drain the fat from the pan, transfer the meat to a plate lined with paper towels, and blot the top of the meat with more paper towels. Then put the meat in a strainer and rinse it with hot water before eating it.

getting wild

Most of us grew up on domestic meat sources like beef, pork, and lamb, but more "wild" meats like venison, buffalo, and elk are being eaten today. These meats are incredibly lean and are available, more and more, in markets around the country as well as in many restaurants. Some game has less fat than skinless chicken breast, yet, like beef, game meats offer high levels of zinc, iron, and other nutrients, as well as protein.

Because it is so lean, game steaks are best served medium rare or rare. Don't over-cook them or they will be tough. However, game is delicious long-cooked in a stew or chili. Game can be an expensive treat if you are not lucky enough to have a hunter in the family for your supply; but if you like it, it's well worth the cost. And with the growing popularity of game meats, you may find a reasonably priced buffalo burger at your local diner! Try one next time.

poultry picks

Poultry such as chicken and turkey are mainstays of a healthy eater's repertoire. Even face to face with the most fattening menu board, you can usually do okay with a grilled chicken or turkey sandwich. (Just be careful of the fat-laden toppings like cheese, mayonnaise, and salad dressing.)

But watch out! Not all poultry is as lean as it is made out to be. Sure, skinless chicken breast and turkey breast are the best in low-fat, high-quality protein. But if you grab a piece of roasted chicken with skin, you could be getting more fat than if you had a steak. You might opt for a turkey burger thinking it is a wise choice, but if the turkey is ground with skin, as it is in most restaurants, you wind up with ten times the fat you bargained for. So make sure you remove the skin from your poul-try, and specifically ask your butcher for turkey ground without skin. When cook-ing, bake, broil, poach, steam, or stir-fry, but keep your bird out of the fryer and away from the gravy, both of which pack on the fat.

While sometimes overlooked by chicken and turkey fans, game birds are extremely lean and often look and taste like red meat. Ostrich, pheasant, quail, and squab are delicious, healthy, and can make for a very special dinner. If you crave duck, choose wild duck, which has only half the fat of domestic duck. Domestic duck and goose are the fattiest of birds, so they should appear on your plate only rarely.

an egg-cellent food

When it comes to protein, don't overlook eggs, one of the most convenient, inex-pensive, nutritious sources of high-quality protein around. They are low in calories and fat and rich in B vitamins, vitamin E, vitamin A, and choline. They are easy to keep on hand and can be whipped up (literally!) in minutes. But because eggs are high in cholesterol (an egg has 213 milligrams of cholesterol, close to the 300 mil-ligrams daily limit recommended by the American Heart Association), they have been stuck on the nutritional hit list for the past twenty years.

comparison chart

FOOD (3OZ COOKED)	TOTAL FAT(G)	CALORIES (G)	SATURATED FAT (G)	CHOLESTEROL	USUALLY, SOMETIMES, OR RARELY
BEEF*					
Top round	3.4	161	1.2	76	U
Eye of round	3.5	136	1.3	59	U
Top sirloin	4.7	153	1.8	76	U
Tenderloin	10.6	194	4.0	72	R
T-bone steak	11.9	196	4.7	50	R
Chuck pot roast	14.4	238	5.6	85	R
Prime rib	28.6	340	11.8	72	R
Ground 95% lean	6	145	2.4	65	U
Ground 85% lean	13	213	5.1	77	R
PORK					
Tenderloin	4.1	139	1.4	67	U
Ham, extra-lean	4.2	111	1.3	40	U
Loin chop, center cut, lean	6.8	171	2.5	70	U
Ribs	18.2	252	6.8	74	R
Shoulder	19.7	280	7.2	93	R
LAMB					
Leg, shank	9.7	184	3.9	76	S
Shoulder	16.2	229	6.8	77	R
Leg, sirloin	16.7	241	7.0	82	R
GAME MEAT					
Elk	1.6	124	.6	62	U
Buffalo	2.0	121	.7	70	U
Venison (deer)	2.7	134	1.1	95	U

FOOD (3OZ COOKED)	TOTAL FAT(G)	CALORIES (G)	SATURATED FAT (G)	CHOLESTEROL	USUALLY, SOMETIMES, OR RARELY
POULTRY[†]					
Turkey breast, skinless	.6	115	.2	70	U
Turkey breast, with skin	2.7	130	.7	76	U
Chicken breast, skinless	3.0	140	.8	72	U
Chicken breast, with skin	6.6	167	1.8	71	S
Chicken thigh, skinless	9.2	178	2.5	80	S
Chicken leg, with skin	11.4	197	3.1	78	R
Chicken thigh, with skin	13.2	210	3.6	79	R
Ground turkey, with skin	11.2	200	2.9	86	R
Ground turkey, no skin	3.2	98	.9	43	U
Domesticated duck, no skin	9.5	171	3.5	76	S
Domesticated goose, no skin	10.8	202	3.9	82	R
GAME BIRDS					
Ostrich	3.2	108	1.2	80	U
Pheasant breast[‡]	3.7	151	1.3	66	U
Wild duck breast[‡]	4.8	139	1.5	87	U
Quail[‡]	5.1	151	1.5	79	S
Squab[‡]	8.5	161	2.2	102	S

[CHART CONTINUES]

FOOD (3OZ COOKED)	TOTAL FAT(G)	CALORIES (G)	SATURATED FAT (G)	CHOLESTEROL	USUALLY, SOMETIMES, OR RARELY
Egg whites(2)	0	33	0	0	U
Egg (1 whole)	5	74	1.5	212	S

*All meat is trimmed to 1/8-inch fat or less, and cooked. Beef is select cut, lamb is choice.
†Poultry is cooked unless otherwise noted.
‡4-ounce portion, raw, without skin.

It turns out eggs may have been unfairly maligned. Doctors now know the cholesterol you eat is not the main factor influencing your blood cholesterol. Eating fat, especially saturated fat, is. So while you want to keep an eye on your cholesterol consumption to be on the safe side, it is far more important to focus on watching your fat intake. Since an egg has just 5 grams of fat (1.5 grams of it saturated), one whole egg a day can fit neatly into a healthy low-fat diet.

But people often tend to eat two eggs at a time, which means 10 grams of fat even cooked without butter. That's close to the amount of fat in that T-bone steak you are supposed to be trading in. And remember, you also have to count the eggs that are in baked goods and other recipes toward your one-egg-a-day limit.

To do eggs right, eat just one—a hard-boiled egg makes an energizing snack or breakfast on the run with a piece of fruit, for instance. You could also stick with egg whites, since all an egg's fat and cholesterol is found in the yolk. But as luck would have it, most of an egg's nutrients are in the yolk, too, so it is a trade-off. I like to split the difference, making my scrambled eggs with one whole egg and one egg white. This compromise works well with many egg-based recipes too, and should help you keep to the suggested maximum of one whole egg a day. And, don't forget, egg substitute is a healthy option, too.

how much meat is enough?

Many diet books on the market today have meat as their centerpiece. But reams of research show that the healthiest diets aren't weighed down with lots of animal protein. Three to six ounces a day (with one egg or two egg whites counting as an ounce) is plenty. See page 237 for the amount of lean animal protein that best suits you.

too much of a good thing?

If protein is so good for you, why not try one of the popular high-protein diets, which promise to help you shed pounds so quickly? First of all, too much protein—more than 150 grams a day—can tax your liver and kidneys. But that is not the biggest problem I have with the most extreme of these plans. The real crux of these diets is that they strictly limit carbohydrates, and as a result ban or severely restrict some of the healthiest foods out there, foods like carrots, bananas, whole grains, and low-fat dairy products. Consequently, they can set you up for nutritional deficiencies and deny your body some of the most powerful disease-fighting foods available. In addition, some are over the top in saturated fat, which has long been linked with chronic disease.

One reason people lose weight so quickly on these plans is that when you severely restrict carbohydrates, you require your body to access its glycogen, or stored glucose, for energy. As you deplete your glycogen stores, you also lose water—3 grams of water goes along with each gram of glycogen. That's why people lose so much "weight" immediately on a high-protein plan—as the body's glycogen stores are burned, you also lose a lot of water. And all that water loss can put you at risk for dehydration and constipation.

Some of the more moderate high-protein plans (those that allow the healthiest carbs, and fats) are probably safe and can lead to sustained weight loss. But from what people tell me, they can get pretty boring, and in the end, all that protein just isn't the healthiest way for most people to go.

recipes

spinach-feta frittata SERVES 4

The combination of whole eggs and egg white gives this frittata a rich texture while keeping it lean. Feta cheese naturally has about a third less fat than other cheeses and adds lots of flavor.

4 large eggs

4 egg whites

2 teaspoons olive oil

1 medium onion, chopped

1 10-ounce package of frozen spinach, thawed and drained of excess water

1/4 teaspoon salt

1/2 teaspoon freshly ground black pepper

1/4 cup feta cheese, crumbled

In a medium bowl, whisk together the eggs and egg whites and set aside.

In a large, ovenproof, nonstick skillet, heat the oil over a medium flame. Add the onion and sauté until it begins to soften, about 5 minutes. Add the spinach and heat for 1 to 2 minutes. Stir in the salt and pepper. Pour the egg mixture over the vegetables in the skillet, covering them evenly. Reduce the heat to medium-low, cover, and let simmer until the egg mixture has set around the edges but is still somewhat liquid in the center, about 8 minutes. Sprinkle with the feta cheese.

Meanwhile, preheat the broiler. Place the skillet under the broiler, about 2 inches from the heat source, until the surface is set and golden brown, 1 to 2 minutes. Be careful not to overcook, or the egg mixture will become tough.

Cut the frittata into 8 wedges and serve.

Calories 148; Fat 7.9 g (Sat 2.2 g, Mono 3.7 g, Poly 1.0 g); Protein 12.5 g; Carb 7.3 g; Fiber 2.8 g; Chol 214 mg; Sodium 336 mg

roasted pork tenderloin SERVES 4 TO 6

This is an easy dish that will please any carnivore.

2 tablespoons low-sodium soy sauce

2 tablespoons olive oil

2 tablespoons orange juice

1 garlic clove, minced

1 teaspoon peeled and freshly grated ginger, or 1/2 teaspoon ground ginger

1 teaspoon freshly ground black pepper

2 pork tenderloins (about 3/4 pound each)

In a large bowl, whisk together the soy sauce, olive oil, orange juice, garlic, ginger, and pepper. Add the pork, cover, and let marinate in the refrigerator for 2 to 8 hours. Preheat the broiler. Place the pork on a roasting pan and broil for 15 minutes, 2 to 4 inches from the flame, turning the meat once at the halfway point.

Calories 159; Fat 6.1 g (Sat 1.6 g, Mono 3.4 g, Poly .6 g); Protein 23.9 g; Carb .5 g; Fiber 0 g; Chol 74 mg; Sodium 157 mg

venison with mushroom-wine sauce   SERVES 4

If you can't get venison, pork tenderloin works very well in this recipe, too.

1/3 cup flour

1/4 teaspoon salt, plus more to taste

1/4 teaspoon freshly ground black pepper, plus more to taste

1 to 1 1/2 pounds boneless venison steak, cut into 1/2-inch-thick slices

1 tablespoon olive oil

1/4 cup chopped shallots

1 garlic clove, minced

1 1/2 cups chopped mushrooms

1 tablespoon tomato paste

1/2 cup red wine

1/2 cup low-sodium chicken broth

Put the flour in a shallow dish and season it with 1/4 teaspoon salt and 1/4 teaspoon pepper. Lightly dredge the venison in the seasoned flour. Heat the olive oil in a large skillet over a medium-high flame. Cook the venison for 2 minutes on each side. Transfer the venison to a plate and cover it to keep warm.

Reduce the heat in the skillet to medium, add the shallots and garlic, and cook for 1 minute, stirring constantly. Add the mushrooms and sauté for about 3 minutes. Stir in the tomato paste. Add the wine and chicken broth, raise the heat to medium-high, and cook for 1 minute more. Return the meat to the pan and simmer until heated, about 1 minute. Season with salt and pepper to taste.

Calories 276; Fat 7.8 g (Sat 2 g, Mono 3.5 g, Poly 1.3 g); Protein 35.5 g; Carb 10.4 g; Fiber .6 g; Chol 121 mg; Sodium 272 mg

beef steak soft tacos SERVES 4

Soft corn tortillas, lean beef, and crunchy cabbage make these tacos especially healthy. They are a breeze to make and fun to eat.

1/2 cup freshly squeezed lime juice

3 garlic cloves, minced

2 teaspoons chili powder

1 tablespoon olive oil

1 1/4 pounds top sirloin steaks, cut 1 inch thick

12 small corn tortillas (5 to 6 inches in diameter)

3/4 cup store-bought tomato salsa

4 cups shredded cabbage

1/2 cup chopped cilantro

1/2 cup chopped scallions

In a large bowl, whisk together 1/4 cup of the lime juice with the garlic, chili powder, and olive oil. Put the steaks in the bowl, turn them to distribute the marinade, cover, and marinate in the refrigerator for 1 hour.

Remove the steaks from the marinade and discard the marinade. Grill the steaks over medium heat for about 12 minutes for medium-rare, turning once. Carve into thin slices.

Place the tortillas on the grill to warm, turning once, about 30 seconds.

To prepare the tacos, place a few slices of meat on a warm tortilla, top with a tablespoon of salsa, 1/3 cup cabbage, 2 teaspoons each of cilantro and scallions, and 1 teaspoon lime juice. Serve open-faced so the diner can fold it himself, or fold and secure with a toothpick.

Calories 426; Fat 10.3 g (Sat 3 g, Mono 4.5 g, Poly 14 g); Protein 40 g; Carb 44.4 g; Fiber 6.7 g; Chol 82 mg; Sodium 324 mg

old-fashioned turkey meatloaf SERVES 8

This meatloaf is just like the family classic, but with 60 percent less fat.

1 tablespoon olive oil

1 medium onion, finely chopped

1 large carrot, finely chopped

1 celery stalk, finely chopped

1 garlic clove, minced

1 1/2 teaspoons salt

1 teaspoon freshly ground black pepper

2 teaspoons Worcestershire sauce

2/3 cup ketchup

2 1/2 pounds lean ground turkey

1 1/4 cups unseasoned bread crumbs

2 large eggs, lightly beaten

1/2 cup chopped fresh flat-leaf parsley

Preheat the oven to 350°F.

Heat the olive oil in a large nonstick skillet over a medium flame. Add the onion, carrot, and celery and cook, stirring occasionally, for about 10 minutes, until carrots are tender. Add the garlic and cook for 1 minute more. Remove from the heat and stir in the salt, pepper, Worcestershire, and 1/3 cup of the ketchup.

In a large bowl, combine thoroughly the contents of the skillet with the turkey, bread crumbs, eggs, and parsley. In a shallow baking pan, form the mixture into a loaf and spread the remaining 1/3 cup ketchup over it.

Bake for 1 hour, or until a meat thermometer inserted in the center reads 165°F.

Calories 286; Fat 5.9 g (Sat 1.5 g, Mono 2.1 g, Poly .6 g); Protein 37 g; Carb 21.1 g; Fiber 1.5 g; Chol 109 mg; Sodium 813 mg

ACTION

Starting this week, choose meats, poultry, and eggs from the "Usually" and "Sometimes" lists (see pages 233–235) and keep servings to 3 to 6 ounces per day.

GETTING FIT
making exercise a lifestyle

Think about it. You spend only a small portion of time actually exercising. Even if you work out for an hour a day (which is much more than most people!), the other 23 hours a day are spent working, eating, sleeping, and performing all the other activities of daily life. By becoming more active during those 23 hours, you increase your fitness level and improve your health without even thinking about it.

more movement, more benefits

Think about someone you know whose physical body and energy level you admire. It may be your neighbor with three children who works fulltime and still finds time to go to the gym and coach soccer. Or maybe it's your coworker who puts in long hours and trains for marathons on the weekends. I'll bet that neither one of them spends much time on the couch watching television. They're active without thinking about it—and all that activity adds up to a healthier lifestyle.

While you can add movement to your life in a variety of ways, doing activities with your friends and family is one of the most enjoyable ways to become more active. I've talked before about the benefits of working out with a partner or buddy, and ways to encourage your kids to become more fit.

People who play sports like tennis, racquetball, and golf often play for the sheer enjoyment of the activity. Sure, they're getting in shape as they play, but the bottom line is that's its fun. Team sports like touch football, volleyball, and baseball are a great way to socialize and stay fit. Sign up for a league or set up a game with your family, friends, or neighbors. The emphasis may be on competition or just on having fun.

everyday activity adds up!

Health experts recommend that most people get at least 30 minutes of moderate exercise every day. But activities like vacuuming, gardening, walking the dog, and climbing stairs can all count toward that total. Everything—from standing up out of a chair to walking down a hall to lifting weights or biking—counts, so try to increase physical activity in little ways throughout the day.

For example, park farther away from the store or take the stairs instead of the elevator when you're running errands. Or up the intensity a bit of whatever you're doing now—even household chores like vacuuming, sweeping, and dusting can be challenging depending on how much effort you expend.

Remember, every bit of activity counts. In 20 minutes, an average 140-pound woman will burn approximately the following calories for these tasks (you'll expend more calories if you weigh more than 140 pounds, fewer if you weight less):

Cleaning/housework: 80 to 90 calories

Cooking: 58 calories

Dancing (moderate pace): 80 calories

Gardening: between 70 and 100 calories

Jogging (11:30/mile pace): 176 calories

Mowing grass with a push mower: 90 calories

Playing Frisbee: 108 calories

Shopping: 80 calories

Swimming: 158 to 210 calories

Typing on a computer: 36 calories

Walking (20:00/mile pace): 96 calories

Walking (15:00/mile pace): 126 calories

Walking down stairs: 120 calories

Walking up stairs: 350 calories

Weight training: 110 calories

move more at work

Even if you have a desk job, you can sneak more activity into your workday. Remember, even short exercise sessions will help strengthen your heart, burn calories, and tone your muscles. Better yet, brief breaks will stimulate your metabolism and give you a natural energy boost. Doing something physical stimulates your body and mind.

Walk away Nothing beats a quick walk to clear your head—step outside for a change of scenery or, if the weather's bad, head for the stairs and walk up and down for a couple of minutes.

Take a dip Sit in a stationary chair with your feet out in front of you. Gripping the edge of the chair and keeping your back straight, slowly lower your body 8 to 10 inches and then return to the original position; it will boost your heart rate and tone your shoulders and triceps.

Do it yourself Run your own errands, no matter how menial. Every time you get up from your desk, you burn a few extra calories and keep your muscles in working order.

Squeeze it Keep a tennis ball or racquetball on your desk, and squeeze it as you talk on the phone—it will increase your hand, forearm, and grip strength and relieve tension as well.

Shrug it off One of the best ways to reduce neck and shoulder tightness is by performing simple shrugs. Stand up with your hands hanging at your sides and lift your shoulders as high as you can before returning to your original position. Repeat 10 times and then slowly lower your head toward your chest and take a deep breath.

Save your gas If you drive to work, leave your car five blocks away from your office and walk the difference. Then increase the distance for longer walking sessions. (If you take the train or bus, just get off at an earlier stop.)

Take the long way When you head to the bathroom or for a cup of coffee, take the longest route possible—or add a few quick laps around the office before you return to your desk.

Tighten your tummy When sitting at your desk, do a few chair crunches. Grasping the sides of your chair for balance, lift your legs and pull your knees toward your chest, then slowly lower them back down. Keep your back straight as you do the crunches; as you become stronger, try to do them without holding on to the chair.

Be helpful Volunteer to carry that heavy box into the office—just be careful not to strain your back. You'll burn a few extra calories and also maintain upper-body strength.

take an active vacation

What's your dream vacation? Lying by the beach sipping a piña colada? Relaxation is great, but that doesn't mean you have to loll about all week. Look for ways to incorporate activity into your vacation and you'll feel better. In fact, active vacations are a growing trend. Some trips offer hiking, biking, or walking group tours; others allow you to kayak, raft, or trek.

Take time to hike through a new park when traveling—even if you're not roughing it, nearly every city offers beautiful new vistas to explore. You're more likely to come home feeling refreshed if you include some physical activity during your trip.

Instead of taking one two-week vacation each year, consider breaking up your vacation time into shorter trips. According to one survey, more than two thirds of all Americans say they need only one to three days to feel restored and relaxed. The majority say seeing new places, being away from work, and doing new or different things lead to a restful vacation, and more than half say exercising gives them energy on vacation.

So, plan to include activity on your next trip. You'll feel better, enjoy yourself more, and keep up your healthy habits on the road as well as at home.

Take the stairs Avoid the elevator whenever possible and opt for the stairs instead. If you work on the thirtieth floor, try getting off on the twenty-fifth floor instead. And if it's only a flight or two, the stairs are quicker than waiting for the elevator anyway.

ACTION

Do one thing each day to increase the amount of activity you get in your daily life. That may mean parking a little farther from your office or taking more frequent stretch breaks at work.

FEELING GOOD

pampering

In the past weeks, you've become more mindful and begun to get in better touch with your inner spirit. But caring for the outside of your body—your physical self—can have positive and soothing effects on the mind and spirit as well.

You already wash your face, brush your teeth, and perform other physical self-care tasks without thinking about it. Taking this a step further lets you care for and reconnect with your physical self. This might be as simple as taking a few minutes at night to moisturize your skin with a favorite lotion, or signing up for a massage once a month.

Do you think spending money on yourself is frivolous or vain? Olivia, a thirty-five-year-old child psychologist, used to feel that way. She never paid much attention to fashion or the way she looked, and felt that things like manicures and facials were frivolous luxuries. Throughout her adult life, Olivia focused her energy on intellectual pursuits. She graduated with her doctorate from a great school and had a thriving private practice in New York City. She gave all her energy and heart to the children she helped. While her career was blossoming, she felt something was missing in her life.

Olivia realized that her life was out of balance. She spent so much time giving to and nurturing other people that she wound up feeling drained. While she was proud of her career accomplishments, she also realized that she didn't feel comfortable with her body. She'd never paid much attention to it, concentrating instead on her mind.

Olivia decided it was time to reconnect with her physical self. One of the things she did was pamper herself by indulging in regular manicures and pedicures. This seemingly small act has made her feel better about her physical appearance. She even carries herself differently and feels more confident and comfortable in her own skin.

"It's a way of treating my body like a valuable asset that I cherish," says Olivia. "It's like wearing nice underwear. Even if no one sees it, you feel special, and it reinforces that you are worthy of good things." Taking time to treat herself has helped Olivia find the balance between giving to others and replenishing by giving to herself.

rub yourself relaxed

Massage is more than just a feel-good practice—it appears to have health benefits, too. While the art of massage has been around for thousands of years, it's now being used to ease stress and encourage relaxation and to treat conditions including sports injuries, insomnia, and arthritis.

Massage does more than relax overworked muscles. It can also improve range of motion, increase lymph flow (which helps the body filter out waste toxins), boost energy, and promote endorphin release, which makes you feel good. (And as anyone who's had a massage will attest: it does feel *good*.)

There are different types of massage techniques. Most Western massages are based on Swedish massage, which uses different types of strokes depending on the purpose of the massage. Deep-tissue massage uses slow strokes and pressure to relieve knotted, tense muscles, while myofascial massage involves gentle stretching to help injuries heal.

In studies, massage has been proven to help reduce back pain, nausea and anxiety, insomnia, and lymphedema (painful swelling due to buildup of fluid). But you needn't have a medical problem to enjoy the benefits of massage. While massage is usually performed with the recipient unclothed (but draped with a sheet or towel) and lying down, you can also enjoy a seated massage where the practitioner will work on you through your clothes.

treat yourself

As our lives get more stressful, so does taking time to relax and slow down. Treating yourself to a massage, facial, manicure, haircut, or pedicure is a wonderful way to take some time to yourself—and improve your physical appearance and your mental outlook at the same time!

You don't need a fat wallet for a relaxing spa experience—you can do it yourself in less than an hour's time. Set out a few ingredients—candles, shampoo and conditioner, bath salts, relaxing music if desired, and thick, comfortable towels—so you'll have everything you need. Let your kids and partner know that you're taking a "spa break" and will be unavailable—or, better yet, do this when you're home alone.

Light the candles and put on relaxing music. Run a warm bath with your favorite bath salts or essential oils and soak for at least 20 minutes. As you soak, you can apply a facial mask and deep-condition your hair. Close your eyes, listen to the music, and imagine all tension flowing out of your body.

When you get out of the tub, picture your stressors draining away with the water. Afterward, take a few moments to rub your favorite lotion on your skin and dress in your favorite pajamas. Take a moment to feel how relaxed and at peace you feel—and for less than five dollars' worth of bath supplies!

ACTION

This week, if you can, take time to pamper your physical body, even in a small way. Schedule a massage or a manicure or simply take time to soak in a bath, or treat yourself to a new aftershave or cologne.

action summary

- Shop to replenish your healthy pantry.
- Eat regular meals and snacks, stopping when you are at a 5 or 6 on the hunger scale.
- Drink enough to stay well hydrated, including at least five glasses of water and a maximum of one sugary drink a day.
- Use healthy fats for cooking, dressings, and spreads.
- Eat two to four servings of fruit and three to six servings of vegetables each day.
- Check the ingredient list on your food labels.
- Get at least three servings of whole grains a day and limit refined grains.
- Eat fish at least twice this week.
- Eat at least one serving of nuts, seeds, beans, or soy each day.
- Record in your journal everything you eat and drink.

GETTING FIT

- Walk for 20 to 40 minutes 3 times at mid- or high intensity.
- Stretch and do strength training and core training 3 times.
- Include a fun element in your fitness program.
- Do one thing to increase the activity in your everyday life.
- Continue to attend a fitness class.
- Note your activity in your journal.

FEELING GOOD

- Do the 5-minute breather or mini-vacation once a day.
- Practice mindfulness.
- Say "no" to tasks you don't want to and don't have to do.
- Keep up your bedtime ritual.
- Do a deep relaxation or meditation exercise at least once.
- Optional:
  Tackle a clutter-clearing project.
  Explore journaling.
  Plan a special time with your partner or family.
  Reconnect with a friend.
  Do something to pamper your body.

WEIGHT _____

THIS WEEK'S CHANGES:

1. **Switch to low-fat dairy.**

2. **Sign up for a fitness event.**

3. **Donate some time to charity**
   (optional).

EATING WELL
dairy done right

Chances are you grew up drinking milk—milk on your cereal, milk at lunch, and a tall glass of milk at dinner. All that milk added up to lots of calcium for growing bones, but did you know that a seemingly innocent glass of whole milk has the same amount of fat as two pats of butter? A piece of cheese the size of your thumb contains the same amount, and a meager half cup of premium ice cream has the equivalent of almost four pats! If you pour whole milk on your cereal, indulge in ice cream regularly, or love to have cheese on everything, you are probably eating more butterfat than you realize. Welcome to Week 12, because now, as your final "Eating Well" change, it is time to skim the fat and switch to low-fat dairy.

When you see the results, you'll be glad you did. Each time you substitute a glass of 1% low-fat milk for a glass of whole milk, you save about 50 calories (and more than 5 grams of fat). Over the course of a year that adds up to a 5-pound weight loss. If you take it a step further and nix the cheese on your daily sandwich, you save another 100 calories and drop another 10 pounds by the end of the year. In case you haven't noticed, between last week's changes and the changes I just mentioned, you could be 20 pounds lighter this time next year—without suffering, dieting, or depriving yourself. And your arteries will thank you, too.

low-fat, high-power

Let's get our terms straight here. When I say *low-fat dairy,* I mean milk or yogurt that is either 1% or fat-free (also known as skim) and low-fat cheeses like part-skim mozzarella, reduced-fat cheddar, or low-fat cottage cheese. Nonfat cheeses are fine too, but I have yet to find one that isn't bland and rubbery, so I don't generally recommend them. The small amount of fat in a reduced-fat cheese makes it a much tastier option. Low-fat buttermilk makes the skinny list, too. Despite its buttery name, it's not made with butter. Rather, it's thick, tangy cultured milk that is delicious for baking and in dressings.

When you cut the fat from dairy, you wind up with a great nutritional bargain—low-fat milk products retain the wealth of nutrients of their full-fat counterparts.

Dairy is an excellent source of protein, and the main source of riboflavin (an essential B vitamin), vitamin D, and calcium in our diets. When you go low-fat, you get all that without a lot of calories. Plus, dairy foods are satisfying and incredibly convenient. There is nothing easier than grabbing a yogurt, pouring some milk on whole-grain cereal, or munching some low-fat cheese and a piece of fruit for a healthy breakfast or snack. Now you can even buy drinkable yogurt smoothies, a nutritious food you only need one hand to eat!

the calcium connection

When most people think "dairy," they think "calcium," and for good reason. One cup of low-fat milk provides 300 milligrams of the mineral, about a third of the Recommended Daily Value of 1000 milligrams. Calcium is an essential nutrient that gives structure and strength to bones and teeth, helps muscles work properly, and has a number of other critical functions. Most of the calcium in our bodies is stored in our bones, which act like a bank, saving and withdrawing the mineral as needed. Your bones have stored almost all they can by the time you reach twenty (that's why consuming dairy products is so important to children and teenagers), although you can still make deposits through your thirties. After that, your goal is to maintain the calcium stores you have accrued to keep your bones strong. If you don't consume enough calcium, your bones must tap their reserves so there are adequate amounts of the mineral in your bloodstream. Over time, this constant withdrawal weakens the bone and can lead to osteoporosis.

Calcium isn't the only factor in bone health. Exercise, like the walking and strength training you have been doing, is essential for building and maintaining bone, as are vitamin D, vitamin K, and vitamin C. And since consuming excessive sodium and animal protein cause calcium to be excreted, avoiding too much salt and large portions of meat can help maintain strong bones. Isn't it good to know that all the changes you have been making the past few months have been helping your bones, too?

Besides healthy bones, there is another incentive to get enough calcium. New research shows that consuming sufficient amounts of calcium can also help you burn fat! Scientists believe calcium may act on the cellular level to help keep the metabolism revved and prevent fat storage. The effect is relatively small, but every little bit helps. Studies also reveal that people who consume adequate calcium, especially in the form of dairy, are more likely to be thinner and have less body fat than those who don't. On top of that, calcium may also help keep blood pressure in check and ease symptoms of PMS.

Remember, though, that while getting enough calcium has many benefits (and most of us don't get enough), it is also possible to get too much, especially with all the calcium-fortified foods available now. More than 2,500 milligrams of calcium a day can lead to kidney stones and other problems. If you top off a few servings of dairy with a calcium-fortified cereal and calcium-fortified juice, you may be overdoing it.

lactose intolerance

For all its benefits, dairy is not good for everyone. Between thirty and fifty million Americans suffer from lactose intolerance, which means their bodies don't produce enough lactase, the enzyme needed to digest lactose, the sugar in milk. Americans of Asian, African, Native American, Jewish, or Hispanic descent are most likely to suffer from lactose intolerance, which produces symptoms including cramps, bloating, gas, diarrhea, and nausea after the eating of dairy products. However, many people with lactose intolerance have some ability to digest dairy products and can comfortably eat *small* amounts of milk, or foods like hard cheeses and yogurt, which are naturally low in lactose. Lactose-free and lactose-reduced milks and lactase enzyme tablets are also available. If you suspect you are lactose-intolerant, be sure to see your doctor for confirmation.

probiotics: the good bugs

You may have heard about the active cultures in yogurt or noticed *contains active cultures* on the label. Those cultures are actually good bacteria called probiotics. Probiotics, what I like to call good bugs, help maintain a healthy intestinal tract by warding off the bacteria that make us ill. Probiotics may also protect against gastrointestinal infections, boost the immune system, and even guard against some cancers.

Yogurt is the most common source of probiotics, but not all yogurts have them. Look for brands that boast "live and active cultures" on their label and look for the names of different probiotic cultures, like *L. acidophilus, bifidus, S. thermophilus,* and *L. bulgaricus* on the ingredient list. Also keep an eye out for other products that are now being spiked with probiotics, including cottage cheese and smoothies. They can help your digestive tract function at its best and may keep you healthy as well!

there's more than one way to get your calcium

Whether you're lactose-intolerant or not, dairy is far from the only way to get your calcium. There are many other calcium-rich foods to choose from, such as kale, bok choy (Chinese cabbage), broccoli, sardines, tofu, nuts and seeds, plus an array of calcium-fortified foods including juices, cereals, and soy milk. See the chart below for the calcium content of different foods.

calcium-rich foods

FOOD	AMOUNT	CALCIUM (MG)
Calcium-fortified cereal	¾ cup	200–1000
Yogurt, low-fat, plain	1 cup	448
Calcium-fortified orange juice	1 cup	350
Milk, low-fat	1 cup	300
Soy milk, fortified	1 cup	300
Sardines	3 ounces	204
Tofu, processed with calcium	½ cup	204
Cheddar cheese, reduced fat	1 ounce	200
Salmon, canned, with bones	3 ounces	181
Mozzarella cheese, part skim	1 ounce	180
Sesame seeds	2 tablespoons	178
Soy beans, cooked	½ cup	130
Almonds	⅓ cup	110
Bok choy, cooked	½ cup	79
Cottage cheese	½ cup	69
Beans, cooked	½ cup	25-65
Oranges	1 medium	52
Kale, cooked	½ cup	47
Broccoli, cooked	½ cup	36

10 ways to bone up on calcium

Want to get more calcium into your diet? While you can always take a calcium supplement, there are a variety of simple ways to increase your daily intake of this important mineral:

1. Cook your oatmeal with low-fat milk instead of water.

2. Get a nonfat latte instead of a plain cup of coffee.

3. Make your hot chocolate with low-fat milk instead of water.

4. Sprinkle sesame seeds on your cooked rice, on salads, or in stir-fries.

5. Dollop plain, nonfat yogurt on your baked potato, instead of sour cream.

6. Dip your vegetables in plain, nonfat yogurt flavored with herbs or onion soup mix.

7. Have a handful of almonds and an orange as an afternoon snack.

8. Top your salad with cubes of marinated tofu.

9. Treat yourself to a glass of vanilla-, strawberry-, or chocolate-flavored low-fat milk.

10. Toss a few handfuls of chopped kale or other dark green leafy in your next pot of soup.

recipes

pita pizzas   SERVES 4

These mini-pizzas are perfect for lunch or a light dinner, and they are faster and healthier than pizza delivery. I used mushrooms as a topping here, but you can use any combination of vegetables. It is a great way to use leftovers. Try peppers, onions, olives, or cooked broccoli or spinach.

4 whole wheat pita breads

1 cup store-bought pasta sauce

1$^1/_2$ cups shredded part-skim mozzarella cheese

1 teaspoon dried oregano

2 cups sliced mushrooms

Preheat oven to 400°F. Slice each pita in half to make 2 rounds. Place the pita rounds, cut side up, onto baking sheets. Spread 2 tablespoons pasta sauce on each round. Sprinkle with cheese and oregano, and top with mushroom slices. Bake for 10 to 12 minutes.

Calories 339; Fat 11.4 g (Sat 5 g, Mono 3.1 g, Poly 2 g); Protein 19.4 g; Carb 43.7 g; Fiber 6.1 g; Chol 25 mg; Sodium 846 mg

stir-fried chinese cabbage with tofu SERVES 4

This quick and savory dish has three calcium heavy hitters—bok choy, tofu, and sesame seeds. One serving provides 340 milligrams of calcium, and it is dairy-free. Serve over rice.

3 small bunches bok choy (a type of Chinese cabbage, about 1 pound)
2 tablespoons canola oil
1 tablespoon peeled and grated fresh ginger
3 garlic cloves, minced

$1/3$ cup chopped scallion
1 pound cooked, marinated tofu cubes (see recipe on page 186, or use store-bought)
2 tablespoons low-sodium soy sauce
1 tablespoon sesame seeds

Cut 1 inch off the bottom of the bok choy and wash the separated stalks. Chop the bok choy crosswise into $1/2$-inch-wide strips.

Heat the oil in a wok or large deep skillet over a medium flame. Add the ginger and garlic and cook for 15 seconds, stirring constantly. Add the scallion and bok choy. Raise the heat to high and cook, stirring occasionally, for 5 minutes.

Stir in the tofu, soy sauce, and $1/4$ cup water and cook, stirring occasionally, until the liquid is reduced slightly and the tofu is warmed, about 2 minutes. Sprinkle with sesame seeds.

Calories 243; Fat 18.6 g (Sat 2.1 g, Mono 7.6 g, Poly 7.9 g); Protein 15.2 g; Carb 8.4 g; Fiber 2.4 g; Chol 0 mg; Sodium 688 mg

hot cocoa SERVES 1

This warming treat is a hundred times more delicious than the powdered, watery stuff you've been drinking. Plus you get 315 milligrams of calcium and all the antioxidants of real dark chocolate.

2 teaspoons cocoa powder

2 teaspoons sugar

1 cup plus 1 tablespoon nonfat milk, heated

Mix the cocoa powder, sugar, and 1 tablespoon milk in a mug and stir until it forms a paste. Add the rest of the hot milk and stir until mixed.

Calories 127; Fat .9 g (Sat .6 g, Mono .3 g, Poly 0 g); Protein 9.3 g; Carb 22.1 g; Fiber 1.1 g; Chol 5 mg; Sodium 132 mg

buttermilk mashed potatoes SERVES 6

Buttermilk gives these mashed potatoes a rich and creamy taste and an extra boost of calcium. No one will believe they are nearly fat-free.

2 pounds thin-skinned potatoes, such as Yukon gold (about 6 potatoes), unpeeled and cut into large chunks

1 cup low-fat buttermilk

Salt and freshly ground black pepper to taste

Place the potatoes in a medium pot, cover with water, and bring to a boil over a medium-high heat. Reduce the heat to medium and boil until the potatoes are tender, 15 to 20 minutes. Drain.

Put the buttermilk in a small saucepan and warm it over a very low heat. Be careful not to let the buttermilk get hot, or it will curdle.

Mash the drained potatoes with a potato masher or fork, or use a hand mixer. Beat the warmed buttermilk into the potatoes with a wooden spoon. Season with salt and pepper to taste.

Calories 126; Fat .6 g (Sat .2 g, Mono .1 g, Poly 0 g); Protein 5 g; Carb 25.3 g; Fiber 2.7 g; Chol 2 mg; Sodium 47 mg

ACTION

Eat two or three servings of low-fat dairy and/or other high-calcium foods each day.

competing against yourself

By now, in this last week of the program, fitness has become a healthy habit. Others around you may have noticed a difference in the way you look while you've noticed how much better you feel. Maybe you have more energy, or you sleep more soundly, or you're able to get more done in the day. This week you'll discover how entering a fitness event can add a new spark to your regular routine.

test your mettle

So, ready for a new challenge? Try signing up for a fitness event like a 5K walk or run. Nearly every community offers a slew of events, especially during the summer. Participating in one is a great way to stay motivated and test your fitness in a fun way.

You say you're not competitive? You don't need to be. Most of the people at fitness events don't stand a chance of winning—they're only competing against themselves. They may have registered to support a cause they believe in (many events are fund-raisers for charities or nonprofit organizations) or they simply wanted to participate in a community event. Take along the family or talk to a friend about doing the event with you. You'll be surrounded by like-minded folk and will reinforce the idea that fitness is now an integral part of your life.

Check the local papers for upcoming events or ask at your local health club or running store—they'll often have flyers and information about fitness events. Choose one that's close to home, and that's a reasonable distance for you to cover. Races of 5K (3.1 miles) and 10K (6.2 miles) are popular, and at this point, walking 3 miles should be no problem. Write the date on your calendar and let people know you'll be participating—there's nothing more motivating than seeing people you know (and hearing them cheer for you!) when you're out on the course.

Consider asking a friend to participate with you—if you can train for it ahead of time, all the better. Having someone along will also help keep you from feeling nervous when you line up at the starting line. Selecting an event that raises money for charity is a way to do something good for the community and for your physical health at the same time.

Dee Sanders never imagined that she would become a marathon walker. Dee, fifty-two, had been very close to her mother-in-law and was heartbroken when she lost her to leukemia five years ago. After her mother-in-law's death, Dee received information cards in the mail about an annual marathon to benefit the Leukemia & Lymphoma Society. She tossed the cards away because, although she was quite fit, walking 4 miles 3 or 4 times a week, she couldn't imagine *running* 26 miles!

Then a friend of hers contacted her. He had cancer and was walking the marathon with his wife, and he encouraged Dee to sign up. Dee hadn't realized that many people walk the race. While 26 miles of walking still seemed like a lot, she felt that she could meet the challenge, especially with the inspiration of her friend and her mother-in-law's spirit to guide her.

The Leukemia & Lymphoma Society Team-in-Training Marathon for Walkers and Runners provided her with a coach and a 4-month training plan. Dee successfully finished the marathon and raised thousands of dollars for the charity. "Once I crossed that finish line, I felt I could do anything," she said.

Since then, Dee has walked three more marathons with her thirty-three-year-old daughter, Tracy. Each time, they've crossed the finish line holding hands. "It brought us really close—even closer than before," Dee says. Today she's a volunteer marathon coach, training and motivating other walkers. Her experience has changed her physically and spiritually. "I gained strength and endurance and improved my self-esteem," she says. "I've met the most positive, motivated, wonderful people, and it makes me feel good I am doing something to help."

Dee encourages everyone she meets to sign up for a charitable walk or other event. "You just have to experience crossing that finish line," she says. "You will never be the same again."

the big day

Once you take the plunge and get involved in an event, you may be surprised at how much fun you have. Like Dee, you may want to turn it into a fund-raising event as well. It's usually more convenient to register for the race before the big day—you can pick up your race number and packet the day of the event. Give yourself extra time to find a parking place and visit the bathrooms. Take a few minutes to stretch and warm up before the gun goes off. Don't be surprised if you feel nervous, but enjoy the sense of anticipation.

Don't start off too fast—it's natural to be excited, but try to relax and settle into your usual walking gait. You can always speed up later. Whether you walk or run, concentrate on your form and on maintaining a good pace—you may wind up winning an age group award without even meaning to!

Afterward, take time to cool down, stretch, and rehydrate. Drink plenty of water and have a light snack if you're hungry. Talk to the people around you or walk back to the finish line to cheer the competitors who are still finishing. (Don't worry—there will be someone behind you, I promise!) Savor the feeling of completing the race—you did it! Look how far you've come in less than three months.

goals are good things

One of the reasons I recommend signing up for a fitness event is that it gives you a goal to train for. Research shows that people who set fitness goals are more likely to stick with their exercise routines and perform at a higher level than those who don't. That's one of the reasons that at the beginning of this program, I had you write down what improvements or changes you wanted to make in your life.

Setting goals also gives you a way to achieve successes along the way, just as you have been succeeding with your weekly changes. And there's nothing more motivating than success. So, if you have built-in small goals that you're working toward on a daily, weekly, or monthly basis, and you achieve those goals, you feel good—and if you feel good, you're much more likely to feel good about what you're doing.

When you set a goal—say, to participate in a local 5K walk or run—it gives you something specific to shoot for and can give your workouts new purpose. When you set the goal, consider where you are now—if you're already walking/jogging 3 miles pretty easily, setting a goal of running a 5K race a month or two from now is reasonable. Deciding to run a marathon three months from now is not.

As you're setting your goals, remember to make them specific and measurable. An objective of "I want to run a 5K under 30 minutes" is more effective than "I want to increase my running speed." This way, you have a way of measuring and tracking your success. Define your goal so that you have a way of measuring it.

While you might focus on the overall achievements you're shooting for, don't forget to break down that goal into smaller objectives that you'll work toward over time. Hitting those smaller goals helps keep you motivated to reach the larger ones. By now, you've learned that even a small goal—like, say, walking 3 times a week (hmmm, doesn't that sound familiar?)—can help keep you on target.

ACTION

Find a fitness event to participate in and sign up for it.

sharing the wealth

Throughout the preceding weeks, you've gotten in touch with yourself and strengthened the relationships with those closest to you—your family and friends. This week, I encourage you to take that concern one step further and consider volunteering.

As a volunteer, you can participate in your community, create new friendships, and improve the quality of the place you live and the lives of others. Yet volunteering doesn't have only external benefits—it's internally gratifying as well. Anyone who has committed time or resources toward a good cause knows the satisfaction and the pleasure such work provides. Studies show that volunteers have higher levels of self-esteem and life satisfaction than those who don't give their time and energy. They may also even live longer.

Volunteering can also teach you new skills and introduce you to talents you didn't know you had. Some volunteers enjoy what they do so much that they wind up taking jobs in a similar field; others like the chance to do something different from their normal jobs. In either case, volunteering is a way of connecting with others and getting in touch with the satisfaction of feeling like you're making a positive difference in the world.

where to start

Maybe you already have an organization in mind that you'd like to support. If you're not sure what you'd like to do, consider your interests. Are you good with kids? Volunteering at your local Y, Boys Clubs, or Girl Scouts is an option. Or consider after-school or in-school tutoring programs—most schools are grateful for help.

If you're handy with a hammer, Habitat for Humanity and other programs can use you to help build houses. If you have business or office skills, nearly any non-profit will welcome you with open arms. The key is to find an activity that you'll enjoy—volunteering should enhance your life.

The amount of time you volunteer will depend on what you want. Would you rather have a regular commitment like delivering Meals on Wheels two mornings every month or do something more sporadic? Some volunteer jobs—being a Big Brother or Big Sister, for example—require a time commitment, but others are one-shot deals.

Still not sure what you might want to do? Think about why you want to volunteer, and what benefits you hope to gain from the experience. What kinds of skills, knowledge, or abilities can you share? What are your greatest strengths? What do you like—and dislike—doing? Do you want to work with other people or by yourself? Would you rather do clerical work in an office or be out interacting with people? How much time are you willing to give? What times would be best for you? Choose something that fits your schedule, your skills, and your temperament.

ACTION

This week's recommended action is to sign up to volunteer for one charitable project or event. Choose a one-time-only experience if you're nervous about committing to too much time at the outset—it can even be the fitness event.

WEEK 12
action summary

EATING WELL
- Shop to replenish your healthy pantry.
- Eat regular meals and snacks, stopping when you are at a 5 or 6 on the hunger scale.
- Drink enough to stay well hydrated, including at least five glasses of water and a maximum of one sugary drink a day.
- Use healthy fats for cooking, dressings, and spreads.
- Eat two to four servings of fruit and three to six servings of vegetables each day.
- Check the ingredient list on your food labels.
- Get at least three servings of whole grains a day and limit refined grains.
- Eat fish at least twice this week.
- Eat at least one serving of nuts, seeds, beans, or soy each day.
- Get three to six ounces of lean animal protein a day.

[ACTION SUMMARY CONTINUES]

EATING WELL (CONTINUED)

■ Get two to three servings of dairy or other high-calcium foods each day.

■ Record in your journal everything you eat and drink.

GETTING FIT

■ Walk for 20 minutes 3 times at mid- or high intensity.

■ Stretch and do strength training and core training 3 times.

■ Include a fun element in your fitness program.

■ Do one thing to increase the activity in your everyday life.

■ Continue to attend a fitness class.

■ Sign up for a fitness event.

■ Note your activity in your journal.

FEELING GOOD

■ Do the 5-minute breather or mini-vacation once a day.

■ Practice mindfulness.

■ Say "no" to tasks you don't want to and don't have to do.

■ Keep up your bedtime ritual.

■ Do a deep relaxation or meditation exercise.

■ Optional:

Tackle a clutter-clearing project.

Explore journaling.

Plan a special time with your partner or family.

Reconnect with a friend.

Do something to pamper your body.

Donate some time to charity.

WEIGHT _____

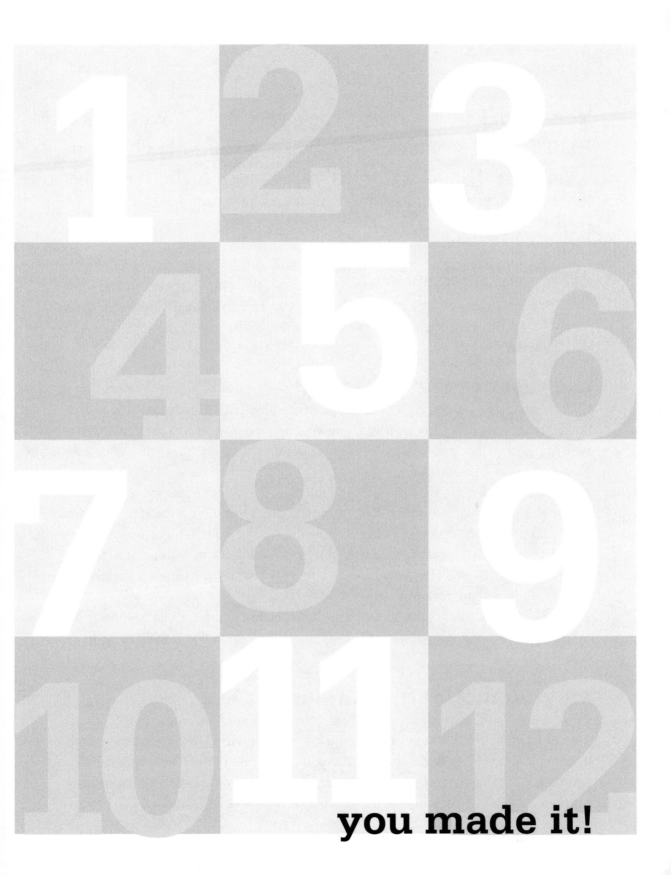

you made it!

You did it! You've reached the end of the 12-Week Action Plan. Take a few minutes and retake the Lifestyle Questionnaire, page 21. I'm sure you'll score much higher on it this time around. Also, remeasure your chest, waist, and hips and note your weight.

Looking at your numbers, and considering how you feel today, ask whether you reached your goals. Where did you improve most? How much weight did you lose? Have you been surprised by how easy it has been to make small changes in your lifestyle—and how they've paid off? Or do you realize there are still some areas you need to improve?

the rest of your life (gulp!)

In some ways, the last twelve weeks has been the easy part. I've shown you how to make small, positive changes in the way you eat, move, and live and have given you the knowledge and template to incorporate those changes into your life. Now . . . you're on your own.

Oooh! Sounds scary, doesn't it? But here's the thing: you've learned a lot in just twelve weeks. You've learned the basics of good nutrition and how to eat to fuel your body and reach your optimal weight. You've discovered how to incorporate movement into your day and created a fitness program that you can maintain or step up to meet your goals. And you've learned how to reduce stress in your life and embrace a more fulfilling, happier lifestyle.

You did all that. I may have shown you the tools, but you put them into practice. Whenever you need to review any of these basic concepts, this book will be here, waiting for you.

staying motivated: a relapse plan

I'm sure there will be times when you find it more difficult to eat nutritiously, to find time to move your body, and to take time for yourself. How do you stay motivated over the long haul? By remembering that you needn't be perfect—every small step you take, every little improvement counts. If you go on vacation and your healthy eating plan goes out the window, pick it up again when you get back home. If work deadlines have kept you from exercising, start again next week. If you're feeling stressed, get back in the habit of doing the 5-minute breather and taking time to decompress regularly.

Remember, at the halfway point, I discussed the importance of a backup plan. Etch this into your mind: it's always better to do *something* for your health—even something relatively minor—than to take no action at all.

If you've completely lost your motivation, however, and even your Plan B seems impossible, use this four-step relapse plan to get back on track:

1. First, cut yourself some slack. Don't call yourself names or beat yourself up because you've "failed." It's counterproductive and only makes you feel worse.

2. Ask yourself why. What's happening in your life to derail your progress? Is it work? Is it your family? Are you overeating to cope with stress or do you feel overwhelmed by the thought of adding even one thing (say, walking) to your day? You have to understand *why* you're now struggling. Retaking the Lifestyle Questionnaire may help you address some of your current concerns.

3. Remind yourself of why you want to make positive changes. You may want to spend some time journaling about this, or write a new letter to yourself about why this is important to you.

4. Make a plan—and stick with it. Even if you only say, "I'll walk for ten minutes after work tonight," that's better than doing nothing. If you've slacked off for weeks, you may want to start from Week 1—or you can jump back into the plan somewhere in the middle.

Some days, it's not easy—you will have times where your plate is filled with more "Rarely" foods than "Usually" ones. You will miss workouts. You will forget to take time to breathe, to relax, to meditate. But as long as you're improving over time, you're also on your way to becoming a fitter, healthier, happier you—all because you've made some small changes in your life.

Small changes really do add up.

appendixes

the **usually/sometimes/rarely** food lists

usually

These foods should be the backbone of your daily diet. Aim to get most of your daily servings from this group.

VEGETABLES

Any vegetables: fresh, frozen, or canned (except those that are fried or in cream sauces)

Vegetable juice

FRUITS

Fruit: fresh, frozen (unsweetened), or canned in natural juice (not sweetened syrup)

100% fruit juice

GRAINS AND STARCHY VEGETABLES

Whole wheat bread, whole-grain rolls, whole wheat bagels

Whole-grain, low-sugar cold breakfast cereals such as Shredded Wheat, Bran Flakes, Cheerios

Whole-grain, low-sugar hot breakfast cereals (for example, oatmeal, Wheatena, brown-rice cereal)

Whole-grain, low-fat crackers (e.g., Wasa crisp bread)

Whole wheat pasta, brown rice, couscous, bulgur, quinoa

Whole wheat or corn tortillas, baked tortilla chips

Whole wheat pretzels, air-popped popcorn

Potatoes, sweet potatoes

Corn

MEAT, FISH, POULTRY, AND EGGS

Fish (anchovies*, catfish, flounder, sole, herring*, salmon*, sardines*, tilapia, freshwater trout, whitefish)

Shellfish (clams, crab, oysters, scallops, shrimp, squid, spiny lobster)

Skinless chicken breast

Skinless turkey breast, ground turkey (no skin)

Top round or eye round select cuts of beef, 95 percent fat-free ground beef

Pork tenderloin, 95 percent fat-free, or extra-lean ham

Game meats: venison, ostrich, buffalo

Egg whites

*Women of childbearing age should limit these fish to two times a month.

BEANS, SOY, NUTS, AND SEEDS
Any beans, lentils, black-eyed peas, split peas, chickpeas
Soy beans; soy products, including soy milk, tofu, tempeh
Nuts: walnuts, almonds, cashews, hazelnuts, macadamia nuts
Peanuts
Seeds: pumpkinseeds, sunflower seeds, sesame seeds, flax seeds
Peanut butter, other nut butters

DAIRY
Skim and 1% fat milk
Nonfat or low-fat yogurt
Nonfat or low-fat cottage cheese
Low-fat buttermilk

FATS & OILS
Olive oil, flaxseed oil, canola oil, peanut oil

sometimes

These foods are more processed, contain more added sugar, and/or more fat than those on the "Usually" list. But it's fine to include moderate amounts of "Sometimes" foods in your diet. Aim to have no more than three servings from this list per day.

VEGETABLES
Cole slaw and other vegetable salads with creamy dressings
Vegetables with cream sauces (such as creamed spinach)

FRUITS
Fruit canned in syrup
Fruit "drinks" or "cocktails"

GRAINS AND STARCHY VEGETABLES
Refined-flour (white) breads, rolls, and bagels
Heavily sweetened cold cereals
Cold cereals that are not whole grain
Crackers that are not whole grain
Biscuits, pancakes, waffles, low-fat and fat-free muffins and cookies
Packaged rice mixes, white rice, regular pasta
Low-fat granola bars, regular granola bars, sports bars, cereal bars
Fat-free cakes, cookies, angel food cake, fig bars, gingersnaps

MEAT, FISH, POULTRY, AND EGGS
Fish (bluefish, cod, halibut, mahimahi, freshwater perch, sablefish, snapper, canned light tuna)
Shellfish (American lobster)
Chicken breast with skin
Skinless chicken thigh
Turkey and ground turkey with skin
Beef tenderloin, sirloin, round tip, bottom round, and pot roast (all trimmed of fat)
Lamb sirloin, lean leg of lamb
Canadian bacon, pork loin (center loin cut, lean)
Low-fat sausage
Whole eggs

DAIRY
Whole milk
Full-fat cottage cheese
Full-fat yogurt
Part-skim mozzarella and ricotta cheese, low-fat cheeses
Feta cheese, Parmesan cheese
Low-fat sour cream, low-fat cream cheese
Frozen yogurt, "light" ice cream, sorbet

FATS AND OILS
Vegetable oil, safflower oil, corn oil
Mayonnaise
Good-quality dark chocolate

SUGARS
Honey, maple syrup, white sugar, brown sugar, molasses
Hard candies

rarely
These foods are highly processed and/or contain a lot of fat and added sugar.
Choose only three servings from this list per week, or less.

VEGETABLES
Fried or battered-and-fried vegetables

FRUITS
Coconut

GRAINS AND STARCHY VEGETABLES

Packaged baked goods and crackers made with hydrogenated or partially hydrogenated vegetable oil

Chips

French fries, fried potatoes

Regular muffins

Pies, cakes, cookies, doughnuts, pastries

FISH, POULTRY, AND MEAT

Fish (grouper, orange roughy, fresh, canned albacore tuna)

Chicken thigh, drumstick, or wing, with skin

Untrimmed beef, lamb, or pork

Regular or "lean" ground beef, corned beef, short ribs, prime rib, chuck blade roast

Hot dogs, turkey dogs, bologna, salami, regular sausage

Regular ham, bacon, pork ribs, pork loin (blade cut, chops, and roasts)

Calves' liver

Chicken liver, duck liver

DAIRY

Full-fat cheeses: Swiss, cheddar, Jack, Brie, etc.

Heavy cream, whipped cream

Sour cream

Crème fraîche

Cream cheese

Ice cream

FATS

Butter

Margarine

Lard and vegetable shortening (like Crisco)

Candy: most commercial candy bars

APPENDIX B
how much should you eat?

First, determine how many calories you need by following these simple steps:

1. Multiply your weight (in pounds) by 15. This tells you the number of calories you need to maintain your weight. (This calculation assumes you are following the activities outlined in this book, or are otherwise moderately active.)
2. Subtract 500 from that number to lose 1 pound a week, or subtract 1,000 to lose 2 pounds a week. (Do not let your caloric intake fall below 1,200 calories per day, however.)
3. If you want to gain weight, add 500 to your maintenance calories.

So if you weigh 150 pounds:

That's 150 x 15 = 2,250 calories to maintain your weight and 2,250 − 500 = 1,750 to lose about a pound a week.

Then find the calorie range that you fall into in order to determine how many servings in each food group you should aim for per day. See the next page for serving amounts. Follow the "Usually/Sometimes/Rarely" lists, pages 233–236, in making your food selections within each group.

FOOD GROUP	I 1,200–1,500 CALORIES	II 1,500–1,800 CALORIES	III 1,800–2,100 CALORIES	IV 2,100–2,600 CALORIES	V 2,600–3,000 CALORIES
Vegetables	3–4	4–5	5	5–6	6
Fruit	2	2–3	3	3–4	4
Grains and starchy vegetables	4–5	5–6	6–7	7–8	8–9
Meat, poultry, fish, and eggs	3–4 oz.	4–5 oz.	4–6 oz.	5–6 oz.	5–6 oz.
Nuts, seeds, beans, and soy	1	1–2	2	2	2–3
Dairy	2	2	2–3	2–3	3
Fats and oils	2–3	3	3–4	3–4	4

At the end of the 12-Week Action Plan, use your new weight to determine your new caloric needs and serving ranges.

serving sizes

Remember, it is okay to have more than one (or less than one) "serving" of a food at a time. Just count it that way.

VEGETABLES (3 to 6 servings per day)

$1/2$ cup cooked or raw chopped vegetable

1 cup raw leafy vegetable

6 ounces ($3/4$ cup) vegetable juice

FRUITS (2 to 4 servings per day)

1 medium fruit: apple, orange, peach, pear, etc.

$1/3$ cantaloupe, honeydew, or other melon (1 cup cubed)

$1/2$ grapefruit

$1/2$ banana

$1/2$ cup canned fruit

1 cup fresh berries

$3/4$ cup fruit juice

$1/4$ cup dried fruit

GRAINS AND STARCHY VEGETABLES (4 to 9 servings per day)

1 slice bread

$1/2$ cup cooked grain (bulgur, oats, etc.), rice, or pasta

$1/2$ cup cooked hot cereal

$3/4$ cup cold cereal

$1/2$ pita pocket

1 medium potato

1 small sweet potato or yam

1 ear corn or $1/2$ cup corn

MEAT, FISH, POULTRY, AND EGGS (3 to 6 ounces per day)

1 ounce cooked meat, poultry, or fish

2 egg whites

1 whole egg

BEANS, SOY, NUTS, AND SEEDS (1 to 3 servings per day)

$1/2$ cup cooked beans, peas, or lentils

$1/2$ cup tofu, tempeh, or soy beans

1 cup soy milk

$^1/_3$ cup nuts

$^1/_4$ cup seeds

2 tablespoons peanut butter or other nut butter

DAIRY (2 to 3 servings per day)

1 cup milk

1 cup yogurt

$^1/_2$ cup cottage cheese

$1^1/_2$ ounces cheese

FATS AND OILS (2 to 4 servings per day)

2 teaspoons oil, margarine, butter, or mayonnaise

2 tablespoons regular dressing

4 tablespoons reduced-fat dressing

Use these visual aids to eyeball serving sizes:

THIS SERVING . . .	IS ABOUT THE SIZE OF . . .
3 ounces of meat, poultry, or fish	A deck of playing cards
1 medium fruit	A baseball
$^1/_2$ cup cooked vegetables, fruit, pasta, rice, or other grain	Half of a baseball
1 medium potato	A computer mouse
1 cup leafy greens	4 lettuce leaves
$1^1/_2$ ounces cheese	4 dice or 1 ice cube
2 tablespoons peanut butter	A golf ball
1 teaspoon fat	The tip of your thumb

sample week of healthy eating

Each day of this sample week adds up to about 1,500 calories. You can use this as a template, increasing or decreasing portions, or adding snacks, according to your caloric needs. Note that this week contains a healthy balance of "Usually," "Sometimes," and "Rarely" foods.

DAY 1

Breakfast	Banana walnut oatmeal (1 cup cooked oatmeal made with nonfat milk, topped with $1/2$ banana and 3 tablespoons walnuts)
Snack	1 hard-boiled egg
Lunch	Minestrone Soup (page 53), with Parmesan cheese (1 tablespoon) Small green salad with Balsamic Vinaigrette (page 102) (1 tablespoon)
Snack	Nonfat vanilla yogurt (1 cup)
Dinner	Roasted pork tenderloin (page 204) Buttermilk Mashed Potatoes (page 222) Steamed broccoli ($1/2$ cup)
	Poached Pears in Red Wine Sauce (page 121)

DAY 2

Breakfast	Cheerios ($1^1/2$ cups) with nonfat milk (1 cup) and sliced strawberries ($1/2$ cup)
Snack	Almonds ($1/3$ cup) and raisins ($1/4$ cup)
Lunch	Grilled chicken breast (4 ounces) over large mixed green salad with Balsamic Vinaigrette (page 102)
Snack	Baby carrots (1 cup) dipped in Mustard Dill Sauce (page 102)
Dinner	Pita Pizzas (page 220) Sorbet ($1/2$ cup)

DAY 3

Breakfast Strawberry Smoothie (page 67)

Snack Apple slices with peanut butter (1 apple with 1 tablespoon peanut butter)

Lunch Turkey sandwich (3 ounces turkey, lettuce, tomato, and avocado on a whole wheat roll)
Vegetable soup (1 cup)

Snack Cookies and milk (2 small chocolate chip cookies and 1 cup nonfat milk)

Dinner Citrus-Ginger Flounder with Snow Peas (page 169)
Brown rice (1 cup)

DAY 4

Breakfast Banana–Peanut Butter Smoothie (page 67)

Snack 1 peach

Lunch Large spinach salad topped with mushrooms, tomatoes, chickpeas, chopped hard-boiled egg whites, and orange slices, with Citrus-Ginger Dressing (page 102), with whole wheat pita bread

Snack Cheese and crackers ($1^{1}/_{2}$ ounces reduced-fat cheese with 5 whole-grain crackers)

Dinner Burger and "Fries" (3-ounce-extra-lean burger on a whole-grain bun with Baked Fries, page 154) with lettuce, tomato, onion, pickle, and ketchup

DAY 5

Breakfast Berries with yogurt, nuts, and honey (1 cup berries, 1 cup nonfat plain yogurt, $^{1}/_{3}$ cup nuts, and 2 teaspoons honey)

Lunch Middle Eastern Platter: Tabbouleh (page 154), hummus, and $^{1}/_{2}$ whole wheat pita with lettuce, tomato, and olives

Snack Cantaloupe ($^{1}/_{2}$) and low-fat cottage cheese ($^{1}/_{2}$ cup)

Dinner Linguini with Shrimp (page 34)
Sautéed spinach (1 cup)

DAY 6

Breakfast   Apple Crunch Oatmeal (page 68)

Snack   Cheese and fruit (1 ounce reduced-fat cheddar and 1 cup grapes)

Lunch   Peanut butter and jelly sandwich (2 tablespoons peanut butter
and 1 tablespoon jelly on whole wheat bread)
1 orange

Snack   Baby carrots (1 cup) dipped in reduced-fat ranch dressing
(2 tablespoons)

Dinner   Small green salad with olive oil (2 teaspoons) and vinegar
White Chili (page 186)

DAY 7

Breakfast   Whole wheat English muffin with
Creamy Honey Walnut Spread (1 tablespoon, page 103)

Snack   Fresh fruit salad (1 cup) topped with nonfat vanilla yogurt
and $1/4$ cup chopped nuts

Lunch   Lentil Soup (1 cup, page 185)
Whole-grain roll

Snack   Hot Cocoa (1 cup, page 222)

Dinner   Lemon-Pepper Chicken (page 33)
Couscous ($1/2$ cup)
Balsamic Swiss Chard (page 119)

supplement recommendations

Supplements cannot take the place of a good diet. We simply don't know enough about all the healthful properties of different foods and how they complement one another to put them into a pill. Besides, I am not a big fan of pills. I don't think people should have to take a handful every day to stay healthy.

That said, I do recommend a simple vitamin regimen that includes a daily multivitamin. A multivitamin acts as an insurance policy so you know you're covering the basics. Even with the best diets, it's hard to get from food some vitamins and minerals in amounts that protect you against disease. Also, several studies show that people who take a multivitamin are healthier overall than those who don't.

Choosing the right "multi" can be a challenge. Many on the market are overloaded with some nutrients and skimp on others. Many also toss in a hodgepodge of herbs and other ingredients that are ineffective and expensive at best, and harmful at worst.

I recommend choosing a vitamin that provides 100 percent of the Daily Value for most nutrients, without any herbal extras. With some nutrients, you may be better off taking less than the Daily Value (iron, for example), and with some, you may want to take more for disease prevention. Below is a list of nutrients and amounts to consider when supplement shopping. It may be hard to find a supplement that fits your needs exactly, but you should be able to find an inexpensive brand that comes close. Of course, if you are pregnant, nursing, or have a medical condition, be sure to consult your doctor before taking any supplement.

NUTRIENT	DAILY VALUE	UPPER LIMIT	RECOMMENDED AMOUNT FOR A MULTIVITAMIN	COMMENTS
Vitamins				
A	5,000 IU	10,000 IU	3,000–5,000 IU	At least 20% should be from carotenoids.
C	60 mg	2,000 mg	60–200 mg	Many multivitamins provide only 60 mg. Consider taking a separate supplement to reach 200 mg daily
D	400 IU	2,000 IU	400 IU	

[LIST CONTINUES]

NUTRIENT	DAILY VALUE	UPPER LIMIT	RECOMMENDED AMOUNT FOR A MULTIVITAMIN	COMMENTS
E	30 IU	1,000 mg	30–400 IU	Many multivitamins provide only 30 IU. Consider taking a separate supplement to reach 400 IU daily.
K	80 mcg	n/a	80 mcg	
B1 (Thiamin)	1.5 mg	n/a	1.5 mg	
B2 (Riboflavin)	1.7 mg	n/a	1.7 mg	
B3 (Niacin)	20 mg	35 mg	20 mg	
B6	2 mg	100 mg	2 mg	
Folic acid	400 mcg	1,000 mcg	400 mcg	
B12	6 mcg	n/a	6–25 mcg	People over fifty should look for a multi with 25 mcg, others should look for 6 mcg.
Biotin	30 mcg	n/a	30 mcg	
Pantothenic acid	10 mg	n/a	10 mg	
Minerals				
Calcium	1,000 mg	2,500 mg	200–1,000 mg	Many multis have no more than 200 mg. Consider a separate calcium supplement to get 1,000 mg daily.
Iron	18 mg	45 mg	0–18 mg	Men and postmenopausal women should take a maximum of 10 mg iron. Premenopausal women can take 18 mg.
Phosphorus	1,000 mg	4,000 mg	0–1,000 mg	Most of us get plenty of phosphorus, and too much can impair calcium absorption. The less in a supplement, the better.

NUTRIENT	DAILY VALUE	UPPER LIMIT	RECOMMENDED AMOUNT FOR A MULTIVITAMIN	COMMENTS
Iodine	150 mcg	1,100 mcg	150 mcg	
Magnesium	400 mg	350 mg (from supplements only)	100 mg	
Zinc	15 mg	40 mg	15 mg	
Selenium	70 mcg	400 mcg	70–200 mcg	Many multis contain only 70 mcg. Consider taking a separate supplement to obtain a total of 200 mcg daily.
Copper	2 mg	10 mg	2 mg	
Manganese	2 mg	11 mg	2 mg	
Chromium	120 mcg	n/a	120 mcg	
Molybdenum	75 mcg	2,000 mcg	75 mcg	

Choline, chloride, potassium, boron, nickel, silicon, and vanadium are often present in multivitmins and are safe but not necessary.

resources

food and nutrition

AMERICAN DIETETIC ASSOCIATION

The nation's largest organization of food and nutrition professionals. The American Dietetic Association (ADA) provides solid nutrition information and can help you find a registered dietitian in your area. (800) 366-1655, www.eatright.org.

ATLANTIC GAME MEATS

This company specializes in farm-raised venison and venison products. www.atlanticgamemeats.com, 1-800-567-4217.

CENTER FOR SCIENCE IN THE PUBLIC INTEREST

A nonprofit nutrition advocacy organization famous for uncovering food and nutrition issues that affect the public. They also provide useful information to consumers and set the record straight on complex issues. They publish the excellent *Nutrition Action Heathletter.* (202) 332-9110, www.cspinet.org.

CONSUMER LAB

A company that objectively tests and evaluates nutrition supplements and other products and supplies the results to consumers. www.ConsumerLab.com.

COOKING LIGHT

An excellent magazine that covers fitness and lifestyle as well as food and nutrition. The recipes are top-notch, and you can access many for free on-line. I also recommend their series of cookbooks. www.cookinglight.com.

EATING WELL

A food magazine with a wealth of high-quality, healthful recipes and insightful coverage of food and nutrition issues. www.eatingwell.com.

ENVIRONMENTAL NUTRITION

An award-winning monthly newsletter that provides sound information on nutrition and health. *Environmental Nutrition* makes sense of all the latest research and gives you the bottom line in a practical, usable way. www.environmentalnutrition.com.

FISH CONSUMPTION ADVISORIES

This website can link you with fish advisories for your area. www.epa.gov/waterscience/fish/states.htm.

HEALTHFINDER

A Web site developed by the U.S. Department of Health and Human Services as a resource for finding government and nonprofit health information on the Internet. It links to over 1,700 health-related organizations. www.healthfinder.gov.

MELISSA'S WORLD VARIETY PRODUCE

Order organic and exotic fruits, vegetables, and other specialty foods on-line or find out where to get them in your area. www.melissas.com, 1-800-588.0151.

SEATTLE'S FINEST EXOTIC MEATS

This company carries an amazing variety of different game meats and poultry. www.exoticmeats.com, 1-800-680-4375.

SHOP NATURAL

A cooperatively run on-line health food store that offers a wide variety of groceries, from whole-grain cereals to nut butters to soy foods, to their members in the Southwest. www.shopnatural.com, 1-520-884-0745.

TUFTS UNIVERSITY NUTRITION NAVIGATOR

This Web site helps you sort through the maze of nutrition information on the Web. It rates the quality and ease of use of hundreds of nutrition-related sites. You can also subscribe to the quality *Tufts University Health & Nutrition Newsletter.* www.navigator.tufts.edu.

USDA FOOD AND NUTRITION INFORMATION CENTER

This Web site gives you access to the National Agricultural Library and provides information about food composition and dietary guidelines. www.nal.usda.gov/fnic/.

fitness

AMERICAN COUNCIL ON EXERCISE

The American Council on Exercise (ACE) is the largest nonprofit fitness certification and education provider in the world. They have numerous fitness publications and reliable information on-line. They can also help you find a certified trainer in your area. 800-825-3636, www.acefitness.org.

AMERICAN VOLKSSPORT ASSOCIATION
A network of walking clubs and organizer of walking events nationwide. 800-830-WALK, www.ava.org.

FITNESS ACCESSORIES
All four of these companies offer a variety of heart rate monitors, pedometers, and other fitness accessories: www.bodytronics. com, www.heartmonitors.com, www.polarheartratemonitors.com, www.cardiosport.com.

ROAD RUNNER SPORTS
This catalog company offers running and walking shoes, gear, and accessories like heart rate monitors, pedometers, and body fat monitors. www.roadrunnersports.com, 1-800-636-3560.

SHAPE UP AMERICA!
A nonprofit, national initiative to promote healthy weight and increased physical activity. The Shape Up America! Web site provides reliable information and tools for healthy eating and fitness. www.shapeup.org.

TITLE 9 SPORTS
This company is geared toward active women. It sells athletic gear, swimsuits, underwear, shoes, sports bars, and accessories. www.title9sports.com, 1-800-342-4448.

THE WALKING CONNECTION
This Web site provides information, products, and services for walkers and hikers. You can read articles pertinent to walkers, find out about walks and hikes in your area, and learn about exciting active vacations. (800) 295-WALK, www.walkingconnection.com.

stress management

THE AMERICAN INSTITUTE OF STRESS
A nonprofit organization that provides information on all stress-related subjects. They have a large up-to-date library of information and a newsletter, and they can refer you to a professional for consultation services. 914-963-1200, www.stress.org.

THE CENTER FOR MINDFULNESS IN MEDICINE, HEALTH CARE, AND SOCIETY

This part of the University of Massachusetts Medical School furthers the practice of mindfulness in the lives of individuals, institutions, and society. It offers a stress-reduction program for individuals. www.umassmed.edu/cfm/srp/.

THE MEDITATION SOCIETY OF AMERICA'S MEDITATION STATION

Use this Web site to learn more about the benefits of meditation and explore different meditation techniques. www.meditationsociety.com.

THE NATIONAL SLEEP FOUNDATION

This nonprofit organization supports the study of sleep and sleep-related disorders. Its Web site includes helpful information for getting better-quality sleep. www.sleepfoundation. org.

contact me: **www.EllieKrieger.com.**

acknowledgments

There are so many remarkable people I'd like to thank for helping create this book. Thank you, Christopher Pavone, my editor, for inspiring me to make a small idea a big reality. I am grateful for all your insight and guidance. Thank you, Jane Dystel, my agent, for being my advocate and keeping everything moving in the right direction. Thanks to the design and illustration team Marysarah Quinn, Jane Treuhaft, and Meredith Noyes for making this book inviting and easy to follow. Thank you, Kelly James-Enger, for being the ultimate professional. I couldn't imagine a smoother collaboration. Thank you, Liz Neporant and Dr. Nadya Swedan, for your expertise in all things fitness, and for being so generous with your time. Thanks to Matthew Jordan Smith, Camille Moonsammy, and Lea Siegal for making me a cover girl. Thank you, Pam Thomas, for helping lay the groundwork. And thanks to all of those who shared their stories and helped with the recipes.

I am also grateful for my family, who has unfailingly supported me and cheered me on. Thanks to my mother and father for teaching me to love food and words, and for encouraging me to go for my dreams. Thank you, Rachelle, my sister, for always being there for me and for all your graphics services. Thank you, Thom, for being my true love and teammate. Lastly, thank you, Isabella, for keeping me in the present while letting me touch the future.

index